MUSCULOSKELETAL
Trauma Simplified

A casebook to aid diagnosis and management

Amna Diwan
Shivani Gupta
R. Malcolm Smith
Robert Perone
Cornelia Wenokor

Musculoskeletal trauma simplified - a casebook to aid diagnosis and management

tfm Publishing Limited, Castle Hill Barns, Harley, Nr Shrewsbury, SY5 6LX, UK.

Tel: +44 (0)1952 510061; Fax: +44 (0)1952 510192

E-mail: nikki@tfmpublishing.com; Web site: www.tfmpublishing.com

Design & Typesetting: Nikki Bramhill BSc Hons, Dip Law, Solicitor

First Edition: © September 2009

ISBN: 978 1 903378 63 2

Printed by Gutenberg Press Ltd., Gudja Road, Tarxien, PLA 19, Malta.

Tel: +356 21897037; Fax: +356 21800069.

Contents

Foreword

As members of the medical community who often deal with bone trauma, we are frequently faced with various clinical and radiographic scenarios in which we are presented with plain films of bones and a contorted extremity on a patient. Often in practice it is a junior doctor who examines the findings of both plain film and patient, sometimes with confusion ensuing. Fracture lines as seen on plain film radiographs are challenging - for the majority of doctors in training, these findings are subtle, confusing and difficult to identify. In the early part of our training, it is demanding to learn the basics of interpretation and management. There are a variety of texts that exist in radiology, orthopedic surgery, and emergency medicine to assist in acquiring such knowledge; however, there lacks a text that provides simple images, matching clinical scenarios, and explanations from which we can begin to form a fundamental base of skeletal trauma. Many junior doctors acquire knowledge in a testing format. However, we have found that a basic review book, written in such a format and targeted towards junior doctors and medical students is lacking. It is our hope that this book will begin to fill that void.

Our book is a simple case-by-case approach to different types of orthopedic fractures. The book is written for the junior doctor, primarily targeted to those in the fields of diagnostic radiology, orthopedic surgery and emergency medicine, and to those residents/registrars in the earlier years of their training when some of the standard textbooks are still too advanced without any basic knowledge. It is also useful for medical students and for practitioners allied to the disciplines listed above.

This book is divided into sections by anatomic location, each containing a number of cases presented as unknowns. Each case contains clinical information, radiographs, a summary of radiological findings and clinical management. The information has been presented in a concise way, giving the required basic information that those interested in musculoskeletal trauma would be expected to know. This allows our readers to test themselves on their ability to identify, describe, and diagnose various types of fractures. Furthermore, they can integrate this information with the standard clinical management involved with that specific disease entity.

This book is essential reading for junior doctors, medical students and for clinicians involved in radiology, orthopedic surgery, and emergency medicine. It is also useful for other physicians who need to be comfortable with reading plain film radiographs and understanding the clinical management. We have taken a unique approach in that we exclusively focus on plain film findings of skeletal trauma, which is a basic required knowledge for practitioners dealing with musculoskeletal trauma.

Amna Diwan MD

Resident, Orthopedic Surgery
Harvard Combined Orthopedic Surgery Program
Massachusetts General Hospital, Boston, USA

Shivani Gupta MB BCh BAO

Resident, Diagnostic Radiology
St Vincent's Hospital and Medical Center of New York
New York Medical College, New York, USA

R Malcolm Smith MB ChB FRCS (Glas) FRCS MD

Associate Professor of Orthopedics
Chief Orthopedic Trauma Service
Harvard Combined Orthopedic Surgery Program
Massachusetts General Hosptial, Boston, USA.

Robert W Perone MD

Associate Professor, Program Director and
Associate Chairman of Radiology
St Vincent's Hospital and Medical Center of New York
New York Medical College, New York, USA

Cornelia Wenokor MD

Assistant Professor
University of Medicine and Dentistry of New Jersey
New Jersey Medical School, Dept of Radiology
Newark, NewJersey, USA

Acknowledgements

This project is dedicated to medical students and junior residents in all fields. We hope it serves as a valuable tool for your understanding of the radiological and clinical aspects of bone trauma. We would like to especially thank our mentors in Boston and New York City, as well as our families and friends for their support while taking on this project. Drs Smith, Wenokor, and Perone: your guidance, knowledge and dedication are what brought this book to what it is today. Thank you for taking the time to clarify, assist and educate. We hope we will someday have the ability to do the same for those training with us. Lastly, but not least, we would like to thank tfm publishing for believing in us and for their unbelievable patience.

Shivani Gupta MB BCh BAO
Resident, Diagnostic Radiology
St Vincent's Hospital and Medical Center of New York
New York Medical College, New York, USA

Amna Diwan MD
Resident, Orthopedic Surgery
Harvard Combined Orthopedic Surgery Program
Massachusetts General Hospital, Boston, USA

Chapter 1

Spine

Case 1

Clinical presentation

A 36-year-old man presents after a high-speed motor vehicle accident. He was a restrained passenger. No air bags deployed in the vehicle. At the scene, the patient was found to have a GCS of 13 due to confusion, but was hemodynamically stable. In the trauma bay, his GCS is improving, but he is complaining of neck pain. He was placed in a hard collar at the scene.

Physical examination

The patient is alert, oriented to person and year, but not to date. He has lacerations on his forehead, and he has peri-orbital swelling and ecchymosis. When you palpate his spine after removing the collar, there is tenderness in the upper midline. You promptly replace the collar. There is no blood on your glove when you remove your hand from palpating his neck. You find no deficits on your neurologic exam.

Review the image below [Figure 1]. Describe your findings.

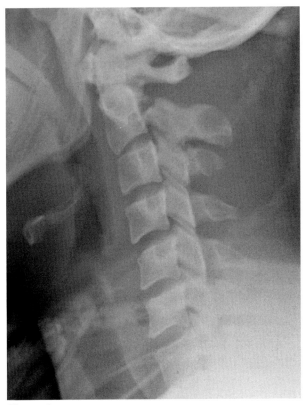

Figure 1.

Questions

1. What is the diagnosis?

2. How do these injuries occur?

3. Describe the commonly used classification system for these injuries.

4. What are other associated injuries?

Radiology findings

A lateral radiograph through the cervical spine demonstrates a mild kyphotic angulation at C2/3. There is a fracture through the pars interarticularis of C2. There is 5mm gapping and 12° of angulation of fracture fragments. There is also malalignment of the spinal laminar line, with gapping between the posterior spinous processes at C1/2.

Answers

1. Hangman's fracture (Type II).

2. In adults, this injury typically results from hyperextension and distraction, as seen in hanging or a high-energy motor vehicle accident (head striking the dashboard). Sometimes in adults and commonly in children, the mechanism is a combination of flexion and distraction as appears to be the case in this example.

3. The classification system proposed by Levine is most commonly used to organize these fractures:
   i) a Type I injury (labeled 'A' in Figure 2) consists of a fracture of the C2 pedicles (pars interarticularis), with the fracture line orientated either vertical or near vertical. There is less than 3mm translation and no angulation. The C2-3 disc space remains intact;
   ii) in a Type II injury (most common subtype), there is greater than 3mm translation and greater than 10° of angulation of fracture fragments. These fractures are unstable and also demonstrate anterior displacement of the C2 vertebral body. There may also be a compression of the anterosuperior corner of the C3 body (labeled 'B' in Figure 2). Type IIa injuries (labeled 'C' in Figure 2) differ from Types I and II because the fracture line is more oblique and there is minimal translation but severe angulation. These injuries also have a different mechanism of injury, as they occur due to a flexion distraction force;

iii) Type III injuries are Type II injuries (angulation and translation) with additional bilateral interfacetal dislocation (labeled 'D' in Figure 2). There is a higher incidence of neurologic deficits.

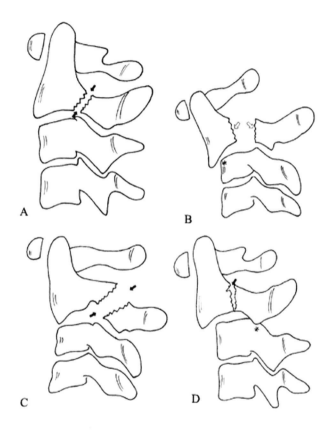

Figure 2. The Levine classification system is pictured; with Type I through III injuries depicted (images A-D, respectively). *Reprinted with permission from Elsevier Ltd. Levine AM, Eismont FJ, Garfin SR, Zigler JE. Spine Trauma. Philadelphia: W. B. Saunders Co., 1998. © Elsevier.*

4. Associated injuries include craniofacial injuries (as seen in this patient), vertebral artery injuries, and cranial nerve injuries.

Management

The stability of this injury depends on the integrity of the C2/3 intervertebral disc.

◆ Type I: cervical collar for up to six weeks.
◆ Type II: requires halo traction, with serial X-rays to verify the reduction. The traction is worn for ~6-8 weeks.
◆ Type IIA: traction is contraindicated, as it may cause exacerbation of this condition. Patients are immobilized in a hard collar.
◆ Type III: while the patient is in the Emergency Room (ER) they should be placed in traction. Definitive treatment will require fixation by fusion of C2 and C3.

Overall, the stability of this injury depends on the integrity of the C2-C3 disc. An MRI can be obtained to further evaluate this. If >50% of the disc is disrupted, the injury is considered to be unstable, and surgical fixation is warranted. (See also the three-column classification by Francis Denis, page 13.)

Key points

◆ Associated injuries include craniofacial injuries, cranial nerve injuries, and vertebral artery injuries. If a patient begins to have nystagmus, vertigo, or complains of blurred vision, a vertebral artery injury should be suspected.
◆ Traction may worsen those injuries classified as Type IIA.
◆ Serial X-rays should be obtained after traction placement to ensure adequate reduction.

References

1. Levine AM, Eismont FJ, Garfin SR, Zigler JE. *Spine Trauma*. Philadelphia, PA: W. B. Saunders Co., 1998.
2. Levine AM, Edwards CC. The management of traumatic spondylolisthesis of the axis. *J Bone Joint Surg [Am]* 1985; 67: 217.
3. Levine AM, Edwards CC. Treatment of injuries in the CI-C2 complex. *Orthop Clin North Am* 1986; 17: 31.
4. Koval KJ, Zuckerman JD. *Handbook of Fractures*, 3rd ed. Philadelphia, PA: Lippincott Williams & Wilkins, 2006: 92-4.

Case 2

Clinical presentation

A 56-year-old man presents to the trauma bay, status post-high-speed motor vehicle collision. He was a restrained driver (positive airbags). The patient was alert and oriented at the scene, and hemodynamically stable. In the trauma bay he is also alert and oriented to person, place, and time, and remains hemodynamically stable. He was placed in a cervical collar at the scene.

Physical examination

The patient is communicative and appropriately answers all of your questions. You find no deficits on your neurologic exam. When you take off his C-collar and palpate his cervical spine, he complains of pain over the bony prominences. You replace the C-collar and the patient is taken to the radiology department.

Review the images below [Figures 3 and 4]. Describe your findings.

Questions

1. What is the diagnosis?

2. How do these injuries occur?

3. How are these injuries classified?

4. If this fracture had not been recognized on initial radiographs, what is the patient at risk for?

5. What should you look for on radiology imaging?

6. What are the risk factors for non-union?

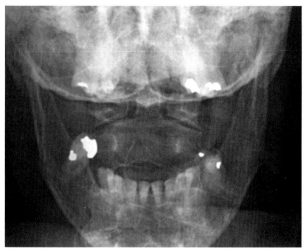

Figure 3.

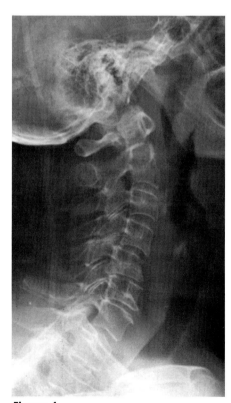

Figure 4.

Radiology findings

An open mouth odontoid view of the craniovertebral junction demonstrates a transverse fracture at the base of the dens. A lateral view of the cervical spine also demonstrates this fracture. There is no significant displacement of fracture fragments. There is slight reversal of the lordosis at C5 and degenerative disc disease at C4/5 through C6/7. Reformatted CT sagittal and coronal images confirm the non-displaced fracture at the junction of the dens and body of C2 [Figures 5 and 6].

Answers

1. Type II dens fracture.

2. Fractures of the odontoid process (dens) occur mostly due to high-speed injuries, such as motor vehicle accidents. In older patients, they can also occur secondary to mechanical falls. Fractures are due to forced flexion or extension of the cervical spine resulting in anterior or posterior subluxation, respectively.

3. Anderson and D'Alonzo classified fractures of the odontoid process into three groups:
   i) Type I fractures are oblique avulsion injuries at the tip of the dens above the transverse ligament. There may be associated occipitocervical instability due to involvement of the alar ligament;
   ii) Type II fractures occur at the junction of the dens and body of the axis (C2 vertebral body) and are the most common type. There may be anterior or posterior displacement, which can be significant;
   iii) Type III fractures extend into the body of the axis.

4. Fractures of the dens are important, because in approximately 10-15% of cases, there is an associated spinal cord injury. Displaced fracture fragments can result in acute spinal cord compression and possible subsequent quadriplegia, and/or death.

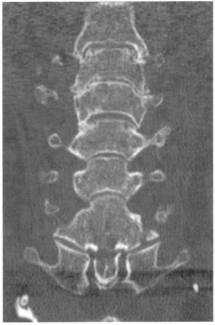

Figure 5. Coronal CT of the cervical spine demonstrates a non-displaced fracture at the junction of the dens and body of C2.

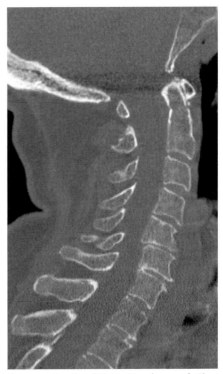

Figure 6. Sagittal CT view of the cervical spine further depicts this Type II dens fracture.

5. When looking for injuries, the lateral c-spine X-ray is usually the most informative but rarely adequately shows the entire cervical spine. CT scanning with multiplanar reformats is now the gold standard. Alignment of the anterior, middle, and posterior spinal columns is important, as there may be abnormal intervertebral disc space widening, abnormal positioning or alignment of spinous processes, retropharyngeal swelling, loss of height of vertebral bodies, or translation of vertebrae.

6. The odontoid peg has a poor blood supply which passes through the bone from the body of C2, and the base of the peg is an area of high stress. These features create the major characteristics of Type II fractures and give them their poor prognosis for healing and a high non-union rate (36%). The risk factors for non-union include age older than 50, more than 5mm of displacement of the fracture fragment, and posterior displacement.

Management

Options for management include stabilization in a collar, application of a halo or surgical stabilization. The latter can involve screw fixation of the odontoid peg or posterior fusion of C1 to C2. A halo may be a reasonable option if the fracture is likely to heal but can be poorly tolerated in the elderly.

Key points

- Fractures of the dens are divided into three groups, depending on the anatomic location of the fracture line.
- It is rare to find neurologic injury with these fractures. Usually, if there is severe cord damage at C2, the patient will be dead on arrival.
- Type II fractures have a high rate of non-union (up to 35%) due to lack of significant cancellous bone.

References

1. Anderson LD, D'Alonzo RT. Fractures of the odontoid process of the axis. *J Bone Joint Surg* 1974; 56: 1663-4.
2. Southwick WO. Current concepts review: management of fractures of the dens (odontoid process). *J Bone Joint Surg [Am]* 1980; 62A: 482-6.
3. Koval KJ, Zuckerman JD. *Handbook of Fractures*, 3rd ed. Philadelphia, PA: Lippincott Williams & Wilkins, 2006: 83-90.

Case 3

Clinical presentation

A 45-year-old man, status post-high-speed motor vehicle collision presents to the ER. He was a restrained driver, and airbags were deployed. He was hemodynamically stable and conversant at the scene, but unable to move his bilateral upper or lower extremities. The patient had to be intubated and sedated en route to the hospital for airway protection. In the trauma bay the patient is in a hard collar, and is hemodynamically stable

Physical examination

The patient has poor rectal tone. His reflexes are hyper-reflexic, he has an inverted brachioradialis reflex, and an upgoing Babinski sign. Once the chaos of the trauma bay has calmed down, the nurse decreases the sedation so you are able to examine the patient. He can follow commands, and he has poor strength in his bilateral upper and lower extremities.

Review the image below [Figure 7]. Describe your findings.

Questions

1. What is the diagnosis?

2. What structures are involved?

3. What type of cord injury is likely to be present?

4. What is your acute management of this patient?

5. What are the four types of incomplete cord injuries?

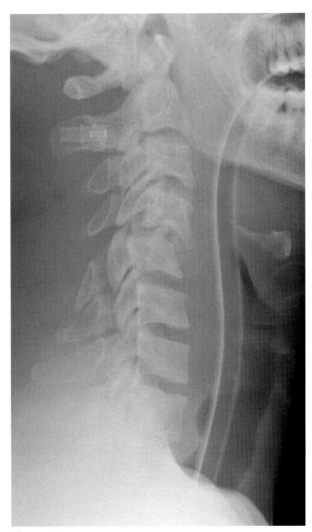

Figure 7.

Radiology findings

A lateral radiograph of the cervical spine demonstrates focal kyphosis and marked anterolisthesis of C4 on C5 (approximately Grade II to III), with a unilateral jumped facet and perched facet on the other side at the C4-C5 level. A CT of the cervical spine with sagittal reconstructions [Figures 8 and 9] further demonstrates the anterolisthesis, and a subsequent sagittal T2-weighted MR image reveals severe narrowing of the spinal canal at this level, resulting in acute cord compression and angulation of the cord [Figure 10].

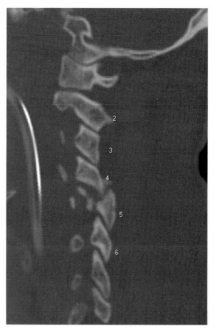

Figure 9. A reconstructed CT image shows facet dislocation (jumped facet) with the inferior facets of C4 located anterior to the superior facets of C5.

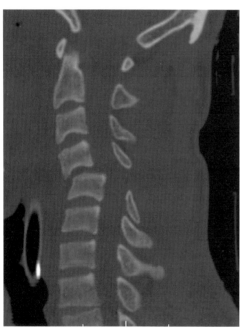

Figure 8. Sagittal CT reconstruction demonstrating marked anterolisthesis of C4 on C5.

Answers

1. Acute hyperflexion injury consisting of a unilateral perched facet and unilateral facet dislocation, anterolisthesis of C4 on C5, and acute cord compression.

2. Such a dislocation involves possible disruption of a variety of structures, including the posterior ligament complex, the posterior longitudinal ligament, the intervertebral disc, and the

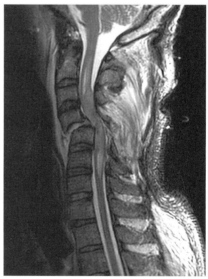

Figure 10. Sagittal T2-weighted MR image further depicts anterior subluxation of C4 on C5, as well as disruption of the anterior and posterior longitudinal ligaments. There is a deformity and angulation of the spinal cord, and resultant acute cord compression. The spinal cord shows increased T2 signal extending from C2 to C6 secondary to hemorrhage and edema.

anterior longitudinal ligament. The result is marked anterolisthesis at the affected vertebral level. The inferior facet of the involved vertebra lies anterior to the superior facet of the vertebra immediately below. This is best appreciated on sagittal reconstructed images.

3. This patient is suffering from an acute cord compression involving nearly the entire cervical spine as seen on MRI, and on physical exam findings. The patient also has a unifacet dislocation, with one perched facet. He will likely exhibit upper motor neuron signs of injury, such as hyper-reflexia, an up-going Babinski's reflex, poor rectal tone, and poor to no motor strength. This patient is intubated, as injury at C4/5 can cause injury to the phrenic nerve, which controls diaphragmatic motion and results in respiratory depression.

4. This fracture needs to be reduced in the ER. Gardner-Wells tongs and cervical traction are used to reduce the fracture.

5. There are four types of incomplete cord injury:
   i)   anterior cord injuries: these have the worst prognosis. Patients have lower extremity weakness greater than upper extremity weakness, pain and temperature sensation loss below the level of injury, and intact proprioception and vibratory sensation. The patient may also display upper motor neuron signs such as hyper-reflexia, and an up-going Babinski's reflex;
   ii) central cord injuries: these are the most common. They are a hyperextension injury, often seen in the elderly after a fall. In this injury upper extremity weakness is greater than lower extremity weakness, upper extremities have decreased sensation compared with lower extremities, and can be hyper-reflexic compared with lower extremities, and sacral sensation is intact;
   iii) posterior cord injuries: these are rare. The posterior column of the cord is affected, and the patient will have loss of position sense below the level of the lesion, but preserved motor and pain sensation;

   iv) Brown-Sequard syndrome: this is a complete hemisection of the spinal cord. The patient will have ipsilateral loss of vibration sensation and motor strength, and contralateral loss of pain and temperature sensation. This lesion has the best prognosis.

Management

The fracture requires acute reduction. This can be done using Gardner-Wells tongs and applied cervical traction. The tongs are applied approximately one finger's width above the pinna of the ear. Anterior displacement of the tongs can help provide more of an extension force; posterior displacement of the tongs can provide more of a flexion force. Since the above is a hyperflexion injury, applying the tongs slightly anterior to provide extension can aid in the reduction. Serial X-rays need to be taken as weights are applied to make sure that the fracture is being reduced. The patient may require open reduction, and will eventually require definitive fixation by fusion of C4/5.

Key points

- Bifacetal dislocation is an unstable injury and has a high association of cord compression and/or damage. These can often be devastating injuries.
- There are four types of incomplete cord injury. The Brown-Sequard syndrome is a complete hemisection of the spinal cord. This lesion has the best prognosis.

References

1. White AA, Johnson RM, Panjabi MD, et al. Biomedical analysis of clinical instability in the cervical spine. Clin Orthop 1975; 109: 85.
2. Selecki BR, Williams HBL. Injuries to the cervical spine and cord in man. Australian Medical Association, Mervyn Archdall

Medical Monograph No. 7. New South Wales: Australian Medical Publishing, 1970.

3. Beatson TR. Fractures and dislocations of the cervical spine. *J Bone Joint Surg* 1963; 45B: 21.

4. Young JWR. The laminar space in the diagnosis of rotational flexion injuries of the cervical spine. *AJR Am J Roentgenol* 1989; 152: 103-7.

5. Rogers LF. *Radiology of Skeletal Trauma*, 2nd ed. New York, NY: Churchill-Livingston, Inc., 1992: 499-506.

6. Koval KJ, Zuckerman JD. *Handbook of Fractures*, 3rd ed. Philadelphia, PA: Lippincott Williams & Wilkins, 2006: 94-100.

7. Thompson JC. *Netter's Concise Atlas of Orthopaedic Anatomy*. Teterboro, New Jersey: Icon Learning Systems LLC, a subsidiary of MediMedia USA, Inc., 2004: 12-20.

8. Bucholz RW, Heckman JD, Court-Brown CM, *et al*. *Rockwood and Green's Fractures in Adults*, 6th ed. Philadelphia, PA: Lippincott Williams & Wilkins, 2006.

Case 4

Clinical presentation

A 56-year-old man presents after a fall from an elevated deck. At the scene he was unable to recall the exact events surrounding his fall, but was otherwise alert and oriented. He has remained hemodynamically stable. He is brought to the ER, and in the trauma bay he is also alert and oriented and hemodynamically stable. He is complaining of low back pain but is found to have intact gross movement and sensation in the lower limbs.

Physical examination

The patient is lying supine on the back board, and he is conversant and appropriately answering all questions. His neurological examination is grossly intact. He is log-rolled and is found to have tenderness in the lumbar spine region. There is no bruising noted, no lacerations, and no step offs. He has good rectal tone. On detailed neurologic examination, he is found to have weakness with hip abduction, and decreased sensation over the proximal thigh but is fully intact distally.

Review the images below [Figures 11 and 12]. Describe your findings.

Questions

1. What is the diagnosis?

2. What is the mechanism of injury?

3. How are these injuries classified?

4. What complications can arise, both immediately and long-term?

5. Describe the three columns of the spine.

6. What is the importance of mechanical instability of the spinal column?

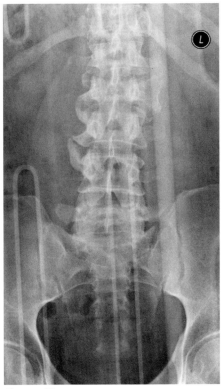

Figure 11.

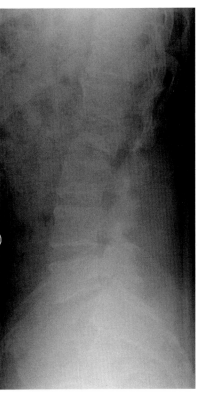

Figure 12.

Radiology findings

On the lateral view, there is approximately 50% loss of anterior vertebral body height of L2 with comminution of the anterosuperior corner of the vertebral body. There is approximately 30% loss of height of the posterior vertebral body height. On the AP view, the L2 vertebra is increased in width compared with L2 and L3. These findings are better appreciated on a CT through the lumbar spine [Figures 13 and 14]. There are fractures involving the anterior and posterior parts of the vertebral body with retropulsion of the posterosuperior portion of the vertebral body into the neural canal. There is significant stenosis of the spinal canal at this level. There is loss of the normal concave contour of the posterior L1 vertebral body. There is complete disruption of the anterior, middle, and posterior spinal columns. These features indicate an unstable injury.

Answers

1. Unstable L2 burst fracture.

2. A lumbar burst fracture is typically seen after a high-energy motor vehicle accident, or a fall or jump from height in which the individual lands on their feet (and also suffers from calcaneal fractures). There is a compressive failure of the vertebral body in all planes with generalized loss of height and widening of the whole vertebrae (seen as widening of the pedicles on the AP view). The axial loading force is transmitted to the intervertebral disc often resulting in retropulsion of the posterior-superior part of the body back into the vertebral canal.

3. Lumbar burst fractures are divided into stable and unstable injuries. A stable injury will not significantly deform under physiologic loads while an unstable injury will. A stable injury will be indicated by a neurologcially intact patient and less than 50% compression of vertebral height. There is often a vertical fracture in the posterior elements, but not a horizontal one. An unstable injury may have a neurologic injury. There is greater than 50% loss of vertebral body height, and there may be a horizontal

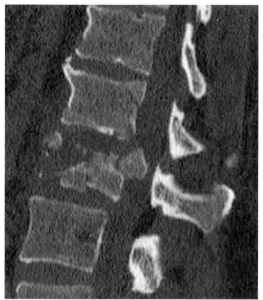

Figure 13. Sagittal CT image through the lumbar spine demonstrates a burst fracture of the L2 vertebral body, with disruption of the posterior cortex and retropulsion of a bone fragment into the spinal canal.

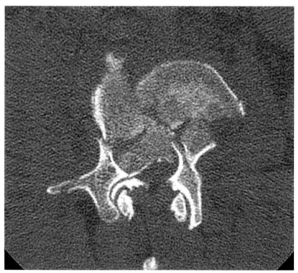

Figure 14. Axial CT image of the L2 vertebral body depicts the degree of comminution of the fracture and the spinal canal narrowing.

fracture in the posterior elements. The Denis classification system is also frequently utilized. In this system, Type A fractures involve both endplates, Type B fractures involve only the

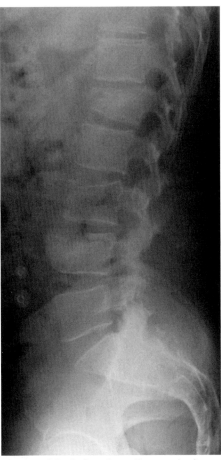

Figure 15. Lateral radiograph in a different patient demonstrates a burst fracture at L1 and anterior wedge compression fractures of L3 and L4.

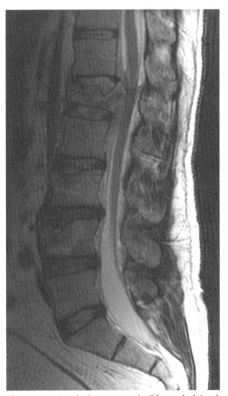

Figure 16. Subsequent T2-weighted sagittal MRI image through the lumbar spine demonstrates a burst fracture of L1 with resultant spinal canal stenosis and cord compression. Compression fractures of the L3 and L4 vertebral bodies are also again identified.

superior endplate (most common), and Type C fractures involve only the inferior endplate. Type D fractures are Type A fractures but with rotation, and Type E fractures are those which demonstrate lateral flexion (resulting in a traumatic scoliosis).

4. Depending on the extent of the fracture, there may be a dural tear. Patients may experience injury to the neurologic system, especially in those cases that have more extensive involvement of the posterior elements. This injury may involve the spinal cord, the cauda equina, or a combination of both [Figures 15-17]. In the long term, patients may suffer from a kyphotic deformity of the spine.

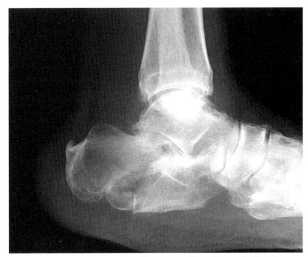

Figure 17. This patient was also found to have bilateral calcaneal fractures.

5. Francis Denis originally proposed the idea of the spine being divided into three columns. The anterior column consists of the anterior longitudinal ligament, anterior part of the vertebral body, and the anterior portion of the annulus fibrosus. The middle column consists of the posterior longitudinal ligament, posterior part of the vertebral body, and posterior portion of the annulus fibrosus. The posterior column consists of the bony and ligamentous posterior elements. The middle column is essential for maintaining stability.

6. Lumbar burst fractures produce a spectrum of mechanical instability of the spinal column. The importance of instability is the risk of associated neurological injury either immediately or developing due to acute spinal stenosis. These injuries usually occur at the level of the cauda equina which is more resilient than the spinal cord so neurological injury is less frequent than would otherwise be expected. There is some relationship between the visible deformity and instability but the energy of injury may be the most important feature causing an immediate neurological injury.

Management

This is an unstable fracture with 50% loss of vertebral body height. The patient has some signs of neurological damage, as he has weakness of hip abduction (L2 distribution) and decreased sensation over his anterior thigh (L1-L3 distribution). Operative fixation of this fracture is indicated. This can be done via either an anterior or posterior approach.

Key points

- Unstable burst fractures are those that involve 50% or more loss of vertebral body height and angulation of 20-30° or a neurologic deficit.
- These injuries can be treated by an anterior or posterior approach, or both.
- The spine can be considered as a three-column structure, anterior, middle, and posterior, initially described by Francis Denis.
- The degree of injury/severity of injury seen on radiographs does not necessarily correlate with the degree of neurologic injury found on physical exam.

References

1. Denis F. The three-column spine and its significance in the classification of acute thoracolumbar spine injuries. *Spine* 1983; 8: 817-31.
2. Bucholz RW, Heckman JD, Court-Brown CM, *et al*, Eds. *Rockwood and Green's Fractures in Adults*, 6th ed. Philadelphia, PA: Lippincott Williams & Wilkins, 2006.
3. Denis F. Spinal instability as defined by the three column spine concept in acute trauma. *Clin Orthop* 1984; 189: 65-76.

Case 5

Clinical presentation

An 18-year-old male wrestler presents to the ER after practice. He reports persistent low back pain, which developed insidiously and has been present for the last three months. He had to stop practice early today because of his back pain and now presents for evaluation.

Physical examination

The patient is a healthy-appearing 18-year-old male. He has pain localized to his lower lumbar spine. There is no radiation to the buttock or posterior thigh, and the straight leg raise test is negative. His pain is exacerbated with hyperextension of the spine. He has a normal heel strike/toe push-off gait. He has minor hamstring spasm bilaterally. There is no scoliosis. There is no tenderness on palpation of his lumbar spine. His distal neurological examination and sciatic tension signs are normal. He reports no bowel or bladder weakness, and has normal peri-anal sensation and sphincter control.

Review the images below [Figures 18 and 19]. Describe your findings.

Questions

1. What is the diagnosis?

2. What is the definition for this type of injury?

3. What classification system is used to grade these injuries?

4. Which spinal levels are most likely to be affected?

5. What is the most likely cause in adolescents?

6. What complications can occur?

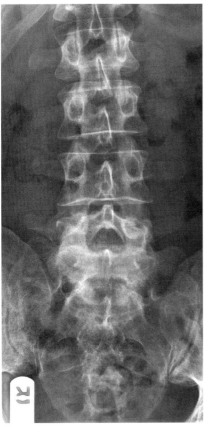

Figure 18.

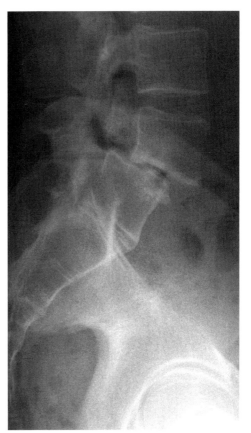

Figure 19.

Radiology findings

Lumbar spine radiographs demonstrate anterior slippage of the L4 vertebral body on L5, known as anterolisthesis. This slippage is classified as Grade II. There is spondylolysis at L4/5, which is visualized as lucency at the pars interarticularis [Figure 20].

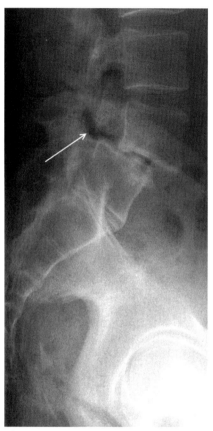

Figure 20. Lateral radiograph of the lumbar spine demonstrates spondylolysis at L4/5 (arrow).

Answers

1. Grade II spondylolisthesis at L4/5 with spondylolysis.

2. Spondylolisthesis is defined as displacement or slippage of one vertebra relative to the adjacent caudal vertebra. The slippage is usually in an anterior direction (anterolisthesis) but may also occur posteriorly (retrolisthesis). It can be associated with spondylolysis, which is when there is a bony defect usually due to a stress fracture in the pars interarticularis developing as a result of excess extension exercise in adolescents. There are two types of spondylolisthesis: dysplastic spondylolisthesis is spondylolisthesis secondary to a congenital abnormality in the lumbo-sacral spine; isthmic spondylolisthesis is spondylolisthesis secondary to a defect in the pars interarticularis, usually a lesion starting as a stress fracture in adolescence.

3. The Meyerding classification of lumbar spondylolisthesis is used, and is based on the degree of anterior subluxation of the superior vertebral body in reference to the inferior vertebral body. A percentage is given to grade the slippage and is relative to the sagittal diameter of the inferior vertebral body:
   i) Grade I is 0-25% slippage;
   ii) Grade II is 26-50% slippage;
   iii) Grade III is between 51-75%;
   iv) Grade IV is 76-100%;
   v) Grade V is anything greater than 100% slippage (spondyloptosis).

   The Wiltse Newman is another classification system used, and more commonly applies to spondylolysis/listhesis in the child and adolescent. This system describes spondylolisthesis based on the likely cause:
   i) Type I is dysplastic spondylolisthesis;
   ii) Type II is isthmic spondylolisthesis and is further broken down into:
   ◆ IIA. Disruption of the pars interarticularis due to a stress fracture;
   ◆ IIB. Elongation of the pars inter-articularis, no disruption. This elongation is due to repeated trauma and healed/healing microfractures;
   ◆ IIC. An acute fracture of the pars interarticularis;
   iii) Type III is degenerative;
   iv) Type IV is traumatic;
   v) Type V is pathologic.

In this case, the patient would be classified as having Type IIA spondylolisthesis based on the Wiltse Newman classification, and Type II based on the Meyerding classification.

4. Spondylolisthesis is most common in the lumbar spine at L5/S1. The second most common affected level is L4/5.

5. In otherwise healthy adolescents, the likely cause is due to repeated stress at the pars interarticularis and pedicle. This results in a stress fracture (the spondylolysis) that may or may not progress to spondylolisthesis. The sports likely to cause such injuries are those involving hyperextension of the spine - which is why this maneuver on physical exam often re-elicits pain. Such sports include, but are not limited to, diving, gymnastics, football and wrestling (such as when opponents are tackled and thrown over each other's backs).

6. If the spondylolisthesis continues to slip forward and cause some compression on the spine, symptoms can result from lumbar stenosis. Such symptoms include radiculopathy, with symptoms related to the nerve root affected, sciatica, and bowel or bladder dysfunction if sacral nerve roots are affected.

Management

If the patient has isthmic spondylolysis and a Grade I slip (0-25%), has isthmic spondylolysis alone without any spondylolisthesis, or has an asymptomatic high-grade slip, this can be treated conservatively, as any other stress fracture in the body. The affecting activity is stopped until symptoms improve. This can take up to 6-12 weeks. The patient is also immobilized in a brace, and physical therapy for stretching and strengthening of the surrounding musculature is conducted. On follow-up, if there is symptomatic improvement the patient is gradually re-introduced into activity. If there is no symptomatic improvement, or if symptoms continue/worsen despite a trail of conservative management, surgical options are considered. Such options include surgery at the appropriate level to repair the pars defect itself (this is done in low-grade slips), or fusion of the level above and below (in high-grade slips).

Patients with dysplastic spondylolysis/spondylolisthesis are treated differently. These patients are at a higher risk of progression of disease and development of neurologic defects. Thus, those with low-grade slips are often frequently examined and fused if symptoms persist. Those with high-grade slips, even if asymptomatic, are often treated surgically because they are at a high risk of progression.

Key points

- Spondylolisthesis is slippage of one vertebra over the adjacent caudal vertebrae, and is most common in the lumbar spine.
- It can occur with or without spondylolysis, a defect in the pars interarticularis.
- There are two types of spondylolysis, isthmic and dysplastic. Isthmic spondylolysis is due to repetitive injury to the pars interarticularis, such as in activities that involve much hyper-extension. Such injuries often respond well to conservative treatment. Dysplastic spondylolysis is due to a congenital pars defect, and is treated more aggressively.
- Spondylolysis and spondylolisthesis are described based on the degree of slippage, as well as the likely cause of the injury. Such descriptions help guide treatment.

References

1. Cavalier R, Herman MJ, Cheung EV, Pizzutillo PD. Spondylolysis and spondylolisthesis in children and adolescents: diagnosis, natural history, and non-surgical management. *J Am Acad Orthop Surg* 2006; 14 (7): 417-24.

2. Khan N, Husain S, Haak M. Thoracolumbar injuries in the athlete. *Sports Med Arthrosc* 2008; 16(1): 16-25.

3. Canale S. *Campbell's Operative Orthopedics*, Vol 3, 9th ed. St Louis, MO: Mosby-Year Book, 1998.

4. Saraste H. Spondylolysis and spondylolisthesis. *Acta Orthop Scand Suppl* 1993; 251: 84-6.

5. Amato M, Totty WG, Gilula LA. Spondylolysis of the lumbar spine: demonstration of defects and laminal fragmentation. *Radiology* 1984; 153(3): 627-9.

Chapter 2

Shoulder girdle and proximal humerus

Case 1

Clinical presentation

A 22-year-old healthy male fell onto his right shoulder while skate boarding. He noticed pain in his right shoulder area after the fall. He iced the area; however, he found no relief. He presents to the ER the day after injury for further evaluation.

Physical examination

He is swollen over the clavicle and tender to palpation. He has pain with a range of motion of his right shoulder. The overlying skin is intact, and there is no tenting of the skin. The patient is breathing comfortably, and distally he has no motor or sensory deficits.

Review the images below [Figures 1 and 2]. Describe your findings.

Questions

1. What is the diagnosis?

2. What is the most common mechanism of injury for these fractures?

3. How are they commonly classified?

4. What is the function of the clavicle?

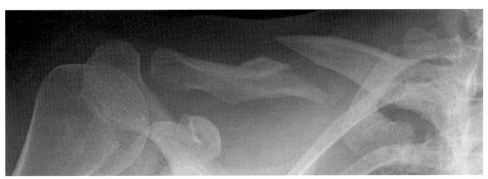

Figure 1.

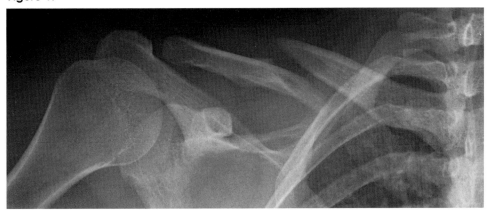

Figure 2.

Radiology findings

There is a displaced fracture of the middle third of the right clavicle. The acromioclavicular (AC) and sternoclavicular joints appear intact.

Answers

1. Mid-shaft right clavicle fracture.

2. Clavicle fractures most commonly occur after a fall onto the ipsilateral shoulder.

3. The Allman classification system is the most commonly used and divides fractures of the clavicle according to the anatomic segment involved. The system divides the fractures into three groups, based on location and anatomy:

   i) Group I (80%): middle third fracture. Upward displacement of medial fragment by sternocleidomastoid muscle. Lateral fragment pulled down by the weight of the limb and gravity;

   ii) Group II (~10%): distal third fracture [Figure 3]. There are three types:

      ♦ in Type I fractures there is no rotation or tilting of the distal fragment because the coraco-acromial and acromioclavicular ligaments are intact;

      ♦ in Type II fractures there is tearing of the coraco-acromial ligament. The medial fragment then displaces superiorly, and the pectoralis major, pectoralis minor, and latissimus dorsi pull down the distal fragment. This creates a deformity. The medial fragment may tent the skin;

      ♦ in Type III fractures the articular surface of the AC joint is involved. Therefore, there is displacement of the articular surface but no ligamentous injuries. This fracture pattern is often confused with an AC joint separation.

   iii) Group III: medial clavicle fractures. These may be associated with other high-grade traumatic injuries at the root of the neck which should be considered first.

4. The clavicle functions as a strut to keep the shoulder girdle away from the chest and protects the brachial plexus, particularly the lower roots, the upper lung, subclavian artery and vein, and beginnings of the axillary artery and vein.

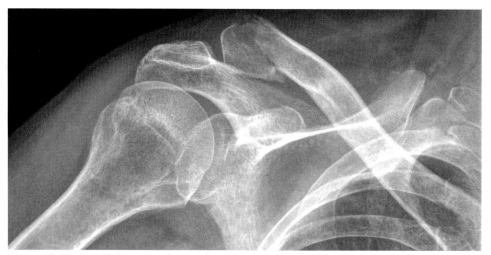

Figure 3. Group II fracture. There is a non-displaced fracture involving the distal aspect of the right clavicle without AC joint or glenohumeral joint disruption.

Management

Most clavicle fractures are treated non-operatively. They heal well but may leave a persistent deformity. Indications for surgery include the following:

♦ Threatened skin or open injuries.
♦ Complex associated injuries such as to the subclavian artery requiring repair.
♦ Marked shortening or medialization of the shoulder girdle - especially if associated with a thoracic outlet problem.
♦ Non-union, which is rare but requires operative repair.
♦ Significant displacement of fracture fragments.

The above indications are not existent in this case. Therefore, the extremity is kept non-weight bearing in a sling until healing becomes evident. Range of motion of the shoulder can begin as soon as comfort allows.

References

1. Allman FL Jr. Fractures and ligamentous injuries of the clavicle and its articulation. *J Bone Joint Surg [Am]* 1967; 49(4): 774-84.
2. Neer CS 2nd. Fractures of the distal third of the clavicle. *Clin Orthop* 1968; 58: 43-50.
3. Neer CS. Nonunion of the clavicle. *JAMA* 1960; 172: 1006-11.
4. Webber MC, Haines JF. The treatment of lateral clavicle fractures. *Injury* 2000; 31(3): 175-9.
5. Koval KJ, Zuckerman JD. *Handbook of Fractures*, 3rd ed. Philadelphia, PA: Lippincott Williams & Wilkins, 2006: 121-6.
6. Thomspon JC. *Netter's Concise Atlas of Orthopedic Anatomy*. Icon Learning Systems Inc., 2002: 5-47.
7. Nonoperative treatment compared with plate fixation of displaced midshaft clavicular fractures. A multicenter, randomized clinical trial. Canadian Orthopaedic Trauma Society. *J Bone Joint Surg [Am]* 2007; 89(1): 1-10.

Key points

♦ Fractures of the middle third of the clavicle are the most common type.
♦ Most fractures occur due to direct trauma to the ipsilateral shoulder.
♦ Based on the above mentioned functions of the clavicle and the underlying anatomy, associated injuries, such as a pneumothorax, damage to the inferior cords of the brachial plexus, damage to underlying subclavian vessels, and associated rib fractures can now easily be identified.
♦ The indications for operating on clavicle fractures are not based on the classification system. Rather they are based on the condition of the skin, complex soft tissue complications, any marked functional impairment and late complications of the fracture such as non-union.

Case 2

Clinical presentation

A 13-year-old helmeted male presents after an accident riding on the back of a motorcycle. He recalls the bike slipping on the road, and him stretching out his left hand to break a fall. He is conscious and hemodynamically stable at the scene and in the trauma bay. An orthopedic consult is called on the basis of left arm pain and swelling, as well as the radiographic findings below.

Physical examination

You notice the patient sitting on his stretcher. Despite his left arm being in a sling, he is holding it close to his body with his right hand. His shoulder is swollen but soft. He can barely lift the arm off the side of his body due to pain. Distally he has palpable pulses, and motor function and sensation are intact. He has no other injuries.

Review the image below [Figure 4]. Describe your findings.

Questions

1. What is the diagnosis?

2. What is the mechanism of injury, and what are some associated injuries?

3. How are these injuries classified?

4. What are the operative indications for this particular injury?

5. What is a floating shoulder?

6. What two normal variants at the shoulder joint can be confused with a fracture?

7. What are the nerves that can be damaged in this injury?

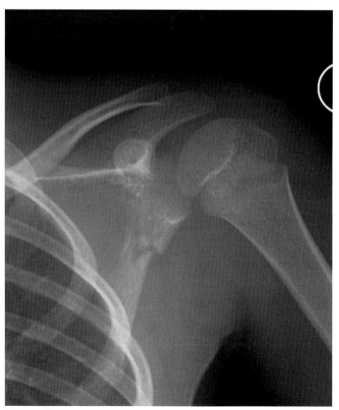

Figure 4.

Radiology findings

There is a slightly oblique fracture extending from the region of the suprascapular notch to the lateral border of the scapula. There is minimal displacement of fracture fragments and no angulation. The articular surface of the glenoid is intact. There is no AC joint separation and no other fractures.

Answers

1. Scapular neck fracture, minimally displaced, not involving the glenoid.

2. Scapula fractures are high-energy injuries, often due to direct trauma in a motor vehicle accident and they are commonly associated with severe chest injuries. Other associated injuries include:
   i) those near the shoulder joint: fractured ribs, fractured clavicle, pneumothorax, brachial plexus injuries, and thoracic spine injuries;
   ii) those associated with high-energy trauma: head trauma, abdominal trauma, pelvic fractures, and femoral shaft fractures.

3. There are multiple classification systems for scapular fractures. The best method is an anatomical classification, describing where the fracture is, whether or not the shoulder joint is involved, and what percentage of the joint is involved. Anatomic divisions include fracture of the scapular body, glenoid, scapular neck, acromion, scapular spine, and/or coracoid. If the glenoid is involved, it is important to note the percentage of involvement of the surface and whether the fracture is comminuted or not, as described above [Figure 5].

4. Surgical indications for a scapular neck fracture include greater than 1cm medial displacement of the fracture fragments, and greater than 40° of angulation.

5. A floating shoulder is double disruption of the superior shoulder suspensory complex (SSSC), resulting in an unstable injury. The SSSC forms a circle, best seen on a lateral view that helps to stabilize the shoulder joint. If looking at the SSSC laterally, going counterclockwise, the components are: clavicle (middle third),

acromioclavicular ligaments, acromial process, glenoid, coracoid process, coracoclavicular ligaments.

6. An os acromiale is an anatomic variant that may be confused with a fracture. It results from failure of one of three ossification centers at the shoulder joint and has a strong association with a rotator cuff tear [Figure 6]. The second

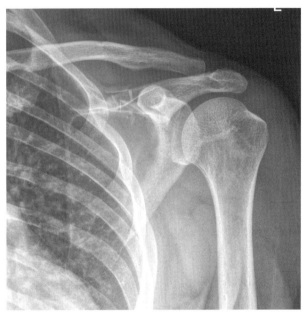

Figure 5. A frontal radiograph demonstrates a comminuted fracture of the superior border of the scapular body, with involvement of the scapular spine.

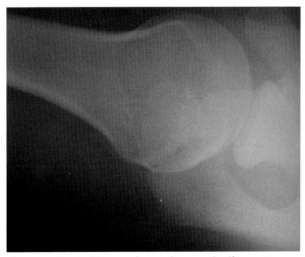

Figure 6. Axillary view demonstrating an os acromiale.

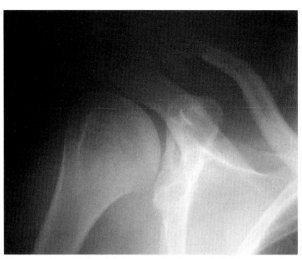

Figure 7. Glenoid hypoplasia, which may be confused with a fracture. There is also a distal clavicle fracture.

anatomic variant that can be confused with a fracture is glenoid hypoplasia [Figure 7]. In cases where it is difficult to tell whether the abnormality is a fracture versus normal anatomic variant, radiographs of the contralateral side are often helpful for comparison. If the anomaly is present on both sides, and only one shoulder is causing pain, it is most likely an anatomic variant.

7. Two nerves that can be injured in a scapular neck fracture are the suprascapular nerve, which runs through the scapular notch, under the superior transverse scapular ligament, and innervates the supraspinatus and infraspinatus, and the axillary nerve, which runs with the posterior humeral circumflex artery through the quadrilateral space, and innervates the deltoid and teres minor muscles. To check the integrity of these nerves based on motor exam is difficult, because patients are often unwilling to move their shoulder secondary to pain from their injury. However, the axillary nerve also provides sensation to the lateral upper arm, and this can easily be tested without causing the patient pain. The suprascapular nerve provides sensation to the shoulder joint itself, which in this injury can be confused with fracture pain, therefore this nerve's sensory exam is not reliable.

Management

The fracture is a minimally displaced fracture of the neck of the scapula, not involving the glenoid, nor any components of the SSSC. This is a stable injury, and can be treated non-operatively in a sling and with early motion as tolerated.

Key points

♦ Scapular fractures are high-energy injuries. As a result they are often present with other high-energy traumatic injuries, particularly chest injury. Additional trauma to surrounding anatomic structures should also be examined.

♦ Normal variants about the shoulder which can be confused with fractures include the os acromiale and glenoid hypoplasia. X-rays of both extremities should be obtained to help decipher injury from anatomy.

♦ Components of the SSSC form a circle that helps to support the shoulder joint. They include the middle third of the clavicle, acromioclavicular ligaments, acromial process, glenoid, coracoid process, and coracoclavicular ligaments.

References

1. Thompson DA, Flynn TC, Miller PW, *et al*. The significance of scapular fractures. *J Trauma* 1985; 25: 974-7.

2. Fischer RP, Flynn TC, Miller PW, *et al*. Scapular fractures and associated major ipsilateral upper-torso injuries. *Curr Concepts Trauma Care* 1985; 1: 14-6.

3. Zdravkovic D, Damholt VV. Comminuted and severely displaced fractures of the scapula. *Acta Orthop Scand* 1974; 45(1): 60-5.

4. Thomspon JC. *Netter's Concise Atlas of Orthopedic Anatomy*. Icon Learning Systems Inc., 2004.

5. Koval KJ, Zuckerman JD. *Handbook of Fractures*, 3rd ed. Philadelphia, PA: Lippincott Williams & Wilkins, 2006: 138-46.

Case 3

Clinical presentation

A 20-year-old college student presents to the ER complaining of severe pain in his right shoulder after a fall while wrestling. He was knocked over by his opponent, landing sideways on his right shoulder, and with his opponent landing on top of him.

Physical examination

The patient is holding his right shoulder close to his body. There is swelling over the top of the shoulder in the region of the AC joint. The skin is intact and there is no tenting of the skin. There is tenderness to palpation over the AC joint, and he has pain with range of motion of his shoulder. Distally, there are no neurovascular deficits.

Review the image below [Figure 8]. Describe your findings.

Questions

1. What is the diagnosis?

2. What is the mechanism of injury?

3. How are these injuries classified? In each group, what radiographic manifestations should you look for?

4. What is the average distance of the coracoclavicular space?

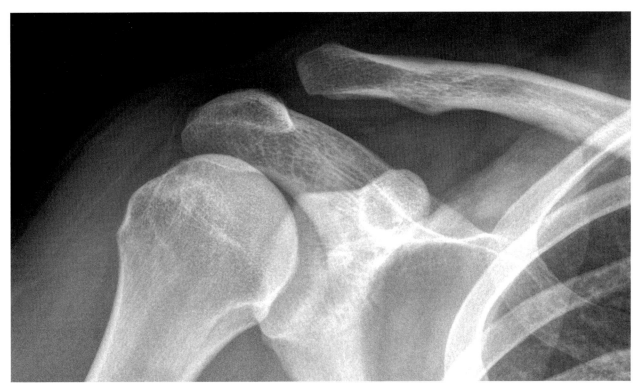

Figure 8.

Radiology findings

There is subluxation of the AC joint space by approximately 13mm. In addition, the distal end of the clavicle is positioned superiorly relative to the medial border of the acromion. There is widening of the coracoclavicular space, measuring 2.1cm. There are no fractures and no glenohumeral dislocation.

Answers

1. Grade III AC joint injury.

2. The most common mechanism of injury is direct trauma to the proximal shoulder. Usually, the arm is adducted, with the force of the trauma hitting the acromion, dislodging it inferiorly from the clavicle.

3. AC joint injuries are classified into six groups.
   i) Type I: tenderness to palpation over the AC joint with no obvious deformity. Radiographs are normal. This is usually a sprain of the AC joint;
   ii) Type II: tenderness to palpation over the AC joint and coracoclavicular ligament with swelling over the AC joint. Radiographs demonstrate subluxation of the AC joint (measuring less than 1cm), without any abnormality of the coracoclavicular space;
   iii) Type III: tenderness to palpation over the AC joint, a step off deformity is sometimes visible, and pain with shoulder range of motion. Radiographs demonstrate further subluxation of the AC joint (now measuring more than 1cm), displacement of the clavicle, and widening of the coracoclavicular space;
   iv) Type IV: tenderness over the AC joint, swelling, deformity noted over the AC joint and distal clavicle, and severe pain with range of motion of shoulder. Radiographs again demonstrate subluxation of the AC joint (measuring greater than 1cm), widening of the coracoclavicular space, and posterior displacement of the clavicle;
   v) Type V: tenderness over the AC joint, swelling, tenting of the skin caused by a superiorly displaced clavicle, and pain with range of motion. Radiographs are similar to that of a Type IV injury, except the clavicle is displaced superiorly;
   vi) Type VI: tenderness over the AC joint, swelling, and gross deformity in that there is flattening of the shoulder. This injury is due to a dislocation of the AC joint, with the clavicle displaced inferiorly. Patients may have damage to the brachial plexus with resultant deficits on physical exam. Radiographs are similar to that of a Type IV injury, except the clavicle is displaced inferiorly (inferior to the coracoid).

4. The average coracoclavicular distance is 1.1-1.3cm.

Management

Most of these injuries can be managed non-operatively. For Type I and II injuries, the patient may be placed in a sling. Range of motion can begin once the patient is comfortable. For Type III injuries, these are also managed non-operatively. However, for some patients the deformity is unacceptable, and some athletes can have pain with extremes of shoulder range of motion. In such cases, surgery may be considered. Types IV-VI are usually treated with open reduction and internal fixation (ORIF) using a compressive screw and/or tendon allograft for reconstruction of the coracoclavicular ligament. These injuries are operated on to alleviate pressure on the skin, and to restore stability about the shoulder joint.

Key points

- The most common mechanism of injury is due to direct trauma to the shoulder.
- These injuries are classified into six types, each with particular findings on physical exam and radiology.
- Types I-III are usually treated non-operatively, whereas Types IV-VI are treated operatively.
- A brachial plexus injury is most likely with a Type VI injury.

References

1. Koval KJ, Zuckerman JD. *Handbook of Fractures*, 3rd ed. Philadelphia, PA: Lippincott Williams & Wilkins, 2006: 127-9.

2. Bucholz RW, Heckman JD, Court-Brown CM, *et al*. *Rockwood and Green's Fractures in Adults*, 6th ed. Philadelphia, PA: Lippincott Williams & Wilkins, 2006.

Case 4

Clinical presentation

A 28-year-old girl presents to the ER with right shoulder pain. During a baseball game, she was sliding into third base, and as she slid, her right arm twisted out and away from her body. She heard a pop, felt immediate pain, and presents for further evaluation.

Physical examination

The patient is uncomfortable. The right arm is in a sling, held away from the body and turned outwards. There is loss of the normal contour of the shoulder, with a palpable round mass anteriorly and inferiorly. Sensation over the lateral arm and lateral forearm is intact.

Review the images below [Figures 9 and 10]. Describe your findings.

Questions

1. What is the diagnosis?

2. What is the mechanism of injury?

3. What are Bankart and Hill-Sachs lesions?

4. If this was an elderly patient, what additional injury should be considered?

5. What is the most common neurological deficit associated with this injury?

6. What is a Velpeau view?

7. What is the apprehension test?

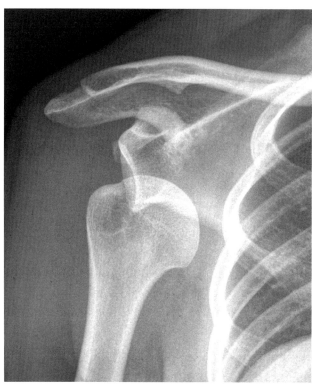

Figure 9.

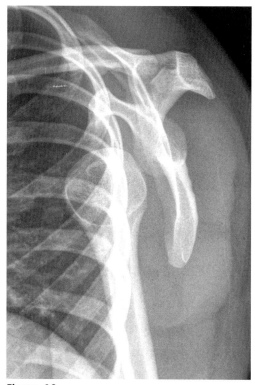

Figure 10.

Radiology findings

There is an anterior dislocation of the shoulder with the humeral head in a subcoracoid position, with marked overlap of the humeral head and glenoid [Figure 9]. On the 'Y' view [Figure 10], the humeral head lies anteriorly and inferiorly to the glenoid.

Answers

1. Anterior inferior shoulder dislocation.

2. The injury occurs secondary to abduction, extension and external rotation of the shoulder joint, as may have occurred above. In adults, the dislocation may be seen after a fall onto the outstretched hand.

3. A Bankart lesion is a tear of the antero-inferior glenoid labrum, and puts the patient at risk for repetitive shoulder dislocations. There may be an associated glenoid rim fracture which is called a 'bony Bankart' lesion [Figure 11]. A

Hill-Sachs lesion is an indentation in the superior and posterolateral humeral head, which occurs as the humeral head anteriorly dislocates and the posterior aspect hits the anterior glenoid rim [Figures 12 and 13]. This lesion can also be identified on plain films and puts the patient at an increased risk for further episodes of dislocation. These lesions are best identified on post-reduction radiographs or CT scans. Injury to the cartilaginous labrum is best evaluated with MRI.

4. In an elderly patient, a rotator cuff tear can be associated with an anterior shoulder dislocation.

5. An anterior shoulder dislocation can result in injury to the axillary nerve, causing weakness and/or paralysis of the deltoid muscle and adjacent sensory loss. The musculocutaneous nerve can also be injured. The musculocutaneous nerve supplies motor function to the brachialis and biceps, and sensation to the anterior lateral forearm. This

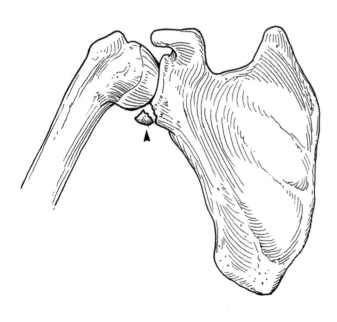

Figure 11. Depiction of a bony Bankart lesion (arrowhead). *Reprinted with permission from the Radiological Society of North America. Hunter T, Peltier L, Lund P, et al. Musculoskeletal eponyms: who are those guys? Radiographics 2000; 20(3): 819-36.*

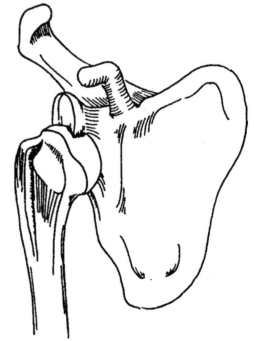

Figure 12. Depiction of a Hill-Sachs lesion. *Reprinted with permission from the Radiological Society of North America. Hunter T, Peltier L, Lund P, et al. Musculoskeletal eponyms: who are those guys? Radiographics 2000; 20(3): 819-36.*

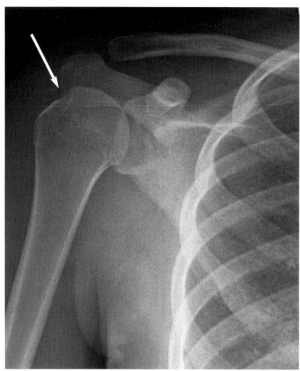

Figure 13. Hill-Sachs deformity of the right humeral head (arrow).

nerve is tested by demonstrating active elbow flexion and by assessing sensation on the anterolateral forearm.

6. A Velpeau view is similar to an axillary view, except the image is obtained from the top of the shoulder, with the camera aimed caudally. This is a helpful view to obtain when it is too painful or inadvisable for the patient to abduct their shoulder for an axillary view. Axillary views are important because they aid in assessing the location of the humeral head in the joint, and the alignment of the humeral head with regards to the humeral shaft. A transthoracic lateral radiograph may also be taken to confirm that the humerus is located in the glenoid.

7. The apprehension test is a test for anterior instability of the shoulder. The patient's affected arm is abducted 90°, and the shoulder is externally rotated. If there is instability, the patient will have the sensation that their shoulder is 'about to pop out,' and they will resist additional motion.

Management

Shoulder dislocations are usually treated by closed reduction and splinting. There are many ways to reduce the shoulder. A good solo method for reducing the shoulder is the Hippocratic technique. In this technique, the operator places one foot in the patient's affected axilla, and applies counter-traction to the affected arm. The foot acts as a fulcrum and the shoulder usually reduces. Post-reduction, the arm should be immobilized for one month in a sling to allow for healing of the anterior capsule. The patient can come out of the sling when comfortable to do gentle pendulums. Following approximately one month of this, the patient may come out of the sling and begin aggressive range of motion with therapy. A major complication of shoulder dislocations is frequent recurrence. The chance of this will be increased if the patient is allowed to mobilize their shoulder too early especially in external rotation.

Operative indications include a failed closed reduction due to interposed soft tissue, an associated displaced greater tuberosity fracture (which will cause rotator cuff dysfunction), and a large glenoid rim fracture (because of a high risk of instability). Recurrent dislocation should be reduced for comfort and referred to a shoulder surgeon for reconstruction. Simple reduction will provide immediate first aid but not produce long-term stability.

Key points

- A Bankart lesion is a tear to the anterior inferior labrum that can occur with dislocation and leads to instability.
- A Hill-Sachs lesion is an impaction fracture, when the posterior lateral humeral head hits the anterior inferior glenoid rim.
- Axillary and musculocutaneous nerves can be injured.
- The most common complication after initial shoulder dislocation is recurrent dislocation, due to damage to the surrounding ligaments, labrum and joint capsule. Young patients are more at risk.

References

1.   Koval KJ, Zuckerman JD. *Handbook of Fractures,* 3rd ed. Philadelphia, PA: Lippincott Williams & Wilkins, 2006.

2.   Bucholz RW, Heckman JD, Court-Brown CM, *et al. Rockwood and Green's Fractures in Adults,* 6th ed. Philadelphia, PA: Lippincott Williams & Wilkins, 2006.

Case 5

Clinical presentation

A 36-year-old man presents to the ER complaining of unremitting shoulder pain for the last 24 hours. He has a history of a seizure disorder.

Physical examination

The patient's arm is in a sling, and he is holding it close to his body. Anteriorly, there appears to be a slight decrease in the rounding of the shoulder joint. Sensation is intact over the lateral shoulder. The patient has pain with attempted range of motion.

Review the images below [Figures 14 and 15]. Describe your findings.

Questions

1. What is the diagnosis?

2. What is the mechanism of injury?

3. What is the main X-ray view that helps you in diagnosing the injury?

4. In reducing the shoulder, what motion should you avoid?

5. List some complications of this injury.

6. Besides trauma, what are other etiologies for this injury?

7. Describe the anatomy of the shoulder internal and external rotators.

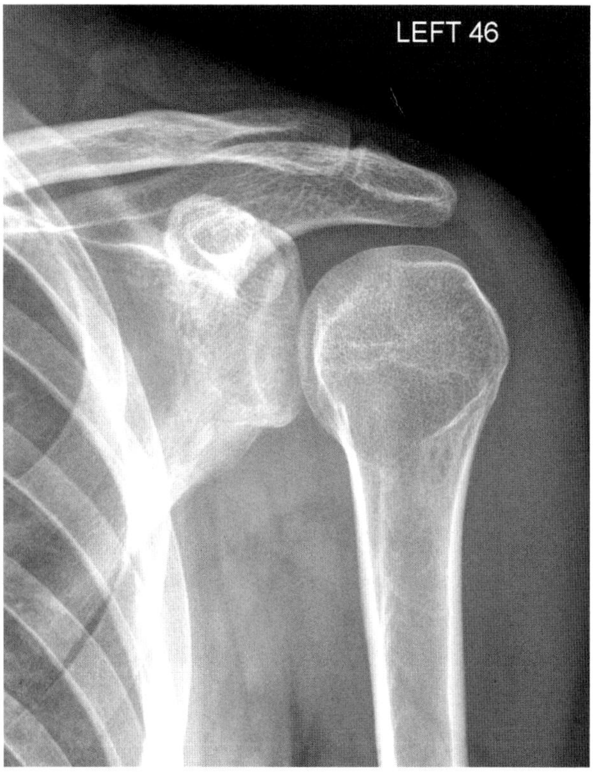

LEFT 46

Figure 14.

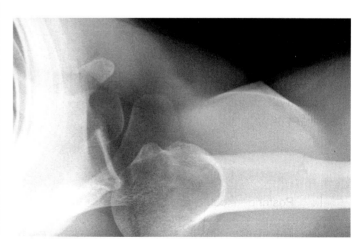

Figure 15.

Radiology findings

Plain film radiographs demonstrate slight overlap between the humeral head and glenoid (tangential views of the glenoid normally demonstrate no overlap). With a posterior shoulder dislocation, the humeral head is displaced medially, causing the abnormal overlap. The humeral head is also fixed in internal rotation (lightbulb sign). The axillary view shows the humeral head lying posterior to the glenoid. There is also a reverse Hill-Sachs lesion [Figure 16]. This is a compression fracture of the anteromedial portion of the humeral head. It occurs due to impaction of the humeral head against the posterior rim of the glenoid and is also known as the trough sign. The trough line describes two parallel lines at the anteromedial humeral head. The first line represents the medial cortex of the humeral head, and the second line represents the margin of the impaction fracture. Another sign to observe is the rim sign (also known as the vacant glenoid sign), which is positive when there is less than 6mm of overlap between the anterior rim of the glenoid and the medial humeral head.

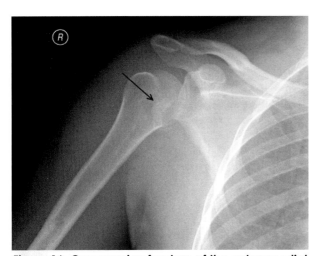

Figure 16. Compression fracture of the anteromedial portion of the humeral head, known as the reverse Hill-Sachs sign.

Answers

1. Posterior shoulder dislocation.

2. The mechanism is axial loading of the extremity combined with internal rotation, flexion, and adduction. In this case, it may have happened to the patient during one of his seizures.

3. The axillary view is the main image that can confirm the diagnosis.

4. During reduction, external rotation of the shoulder should be avoided. The humeral head is stuck behind the glenoid, therefore, external rotation will push it further against the glenoid. The humeral head will remain immobile, and torque will then be applied to the humeral shaft, resulting in a humeral head fracture. However, once the shoulder is reduced, it should be kept in external rotation to maintain the reduction.

5. The patient is at risk for injury to the axillary artery and/or nerve. The patient may suffer from recurrent episodes of dislocations, especially if a reverse Hill-Sachs lesion is present. Patients may also develop post-traumatic arthritis.

6. A posterior shoulder dislocation may occur as a complication of a convulsive seizure. This may be secondary to electroconvulsive therapy or an electric shock.

7. Refer to Table 1.

Management

This injury is difficult to reduce closed. In order to be able to relocate the joint, the humeral head needs to be unlocked from behind the glenoid. The patient should have conscious sedation to relax the muscles as much as possible. Longitudinal traction should be applied to the affected extremity, while the humeral head is pushed down and into the glenoid fossa. Once reduced, the arm is then placed in a sling and swathe or a shoulder spica. This maintains external rotation to prevent redislocation. If the shoulder is unstable and redislocates, or a closed reduction is not successful (which is frequent), the patient should be admitted for reduction under general anesthesia. Once the shoulder is located, it should be immobilized for 3-4 weeks, followed by aggressive physical therapy to strengthen the shoulder internal and external rotators for stability.

Other indications for surgery include a displaced lesser tuberosity fracture or a fracture of the posterior glenoid (which may cause instability and resultant recurrent dislocation).

Table 1. Anatomy of the shoulder internal and external rotators.

	Muscle	Origin	Attachment	Innervation
Shoulder internal rotators	Latissimus dorsi	T7-T12 and iliac crest	Spiral groove of humerus	Thoracodorsal n.
	Pectoralis major	Clavicle and sternum	Spiral groove	Lateral and medial pectoral n.
	Subscapularis	Subscapularis fossa on scapula	Lesser tuberosity	Subscapular n.
Shoulder external rotators	Infraspinatus	Infraspinatus fossa on scapula	Greater tuberosity	Suprascapular n.
	Teres minor	Lateral border of scapula	Lesser tuberosity	Axillary n.

Procedures that are used to reduce a posterior shoulder dislocation include a modified McLaughlin procedure, in which the lesser tuberosity and subscapularis are used to reconstruct a defect in the glenoid and the Boyd-Sisk procedure where the long head of the biceps tendon is used to reconstruct the glenoid defect. If there is extensive damage to the humeral head, a hemi-arthroplasty may be required.

Key points

♦ **Posterior shoulder dislocations (10% of cases) are not as common as anterior dislocations (90% of cases) but are more likely to occur due to seizures or electroconvulsive therapy.**

♦ **Radiographs depict the humeral head lying posterior to the glenoid and may show a reverse Hill-Sachs lesion.**

♦ **During reduction, the arm should not be externally rotated. However, post-reduction, the shoulder should be externally rotated to maintain the reduction.**

♦ **Many of these injuries are difficult to reduce closed, and may require operative intervention.**

References

1. Koval KJ, Zuckerman JD. *Handbook of Fractures*, 3rd ed. Philadelphia, PA: Lippincott Williams & Wilkins, 2006.

2. Perron AD, Jones RL. Posterior shoulder dislocation: avoiding a missed diagnosis. *Am J Emerg Med* 2000; 18: 189-91.

3. Thomas MA. Posterior subacromial dislocation of the head of the humerus. *AJR Am J Roentgenol* 1937; 37: 767-73.

4. Arndt JH, Sears AD. Posterior dislocation of the shoulder. *Am J Roentgenol Radium Ther Nucl Med* 1965; 94: 639-45.

5. Cisternino SJ, Rogers LF, Stufflebam BC, Kruglik GD. The trough line: a radiographic sign of posterior shoulder dislocation. *AJR Am J Roentgenol* 1978; 130(5): 951-4.

Case 6

Clinical presentation

A 56-year-old woman presents to the ER after falling on ice. Her daughter, standing behind her, tried to prevent the fall by holding on to her mother's arm, but the patient still fell and presents in excruciating pain after the incident. Her left arm is held elevated above her head and she is unable to bring it back down to her side.

Physical examination

The patient is sitting in bed with a grimace on her face. Her arm is fully abducted and extended above her head, and her left elbow flexed. There is swelling along her left lateral chest wall, and when palpated, there is round firmness. She reports decreased sensation over her lateral shoulder and numbness and tingling in all of her fingers. She has palpable radial and ulnar pulses.

Review the image below [Figure 17]. Describe your findings.

Questions

1. What is the diagnosis?

2. What is the mechanism of injury?

3. List the potential complications and associated injuries.

4. What is the most commonly injured nerve with this injury?

5. Why should these patients be monitored overnight?

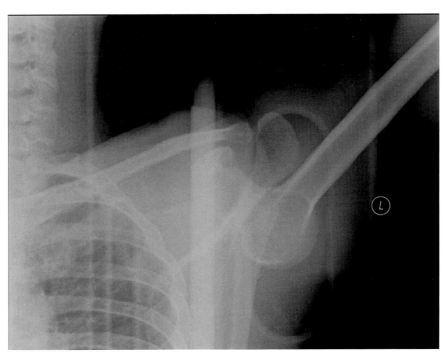

Figure 17.

Radiology findings

There is inferior dislocation of the humeral head, which lies in a subcoracoid position. The humeral articular surface faces inferiorly and is below the glenoid rim. There is no contact between the superior aspect of the humeral head and the inferior aspect of the glenoid rim. No associated fractures are identified.

Answers

1. Luxatio erecta (inferior glenohumeral dislocation).

2. This injury is rare and occurs due to a severe hyperabduction injury of the arm. The humeral neck impinges on the acromion, which levers the humeral head inferiorly.

3. Luxatio erecta is associated with neurological and vascular injuries, including damage to the brachial plexus and axillary artery. Other fractures may co-exist, such as fractures of the acromion, clavicle, humeral head, glenoid fossa, greater tuberosity, and proximal humeral shaft. Rotator cuff injury is also seen. In the long term, patients may experience recurrent episodes of dislocation and shoulder joint instability.

4. The axillary nerve is the most commonly injured nerve in these injuries. Symptoms of numbness and tingling on the 'regimental badge area' on the lateral aspect of the arm indicate a likely injury to this nerve. Recovery is unpredictable and inconsistent after reduction.

5. Although vascular injury to the axillary artery is rare, it can be a devastating complication. If after reduction, there is excessive swelling around the axilla or vascular compromise, a vascular opinion and arteriogram should be performed.

Management

Luxatio erecta can be reduced in the ER. However, since the injury is so rare, not that many orthopedic surgeons are familiar with the reduction maneuver.

The patient should be consciously sedated. Superolateral axial traction is applied by the surgeon, along with countertraction by the assistant. Countertraction is applied by tying a sheet around the patient's body and pulling in the inferolateral direction on the opposite side of the body. As the axial traction is being applied, there is simultaneous decrease in abduction. This should unlock the humeral head from underneath the acromion and allow the joint to pop back into position. Following successful reduction, the arm is immobilized in a sling for 3-6 weeks.

If closed reduction is not possible the patient should be taken to the operating theater. If there is vascular compromise the reduction should be performed urgently in the operating theater, with a vascular surgeon available.

Barriers to closed reduction include intervening soft tissue. This usually involves the inferior joint capsule, as the humeral head buttonholes through it, preventing successful reduction.

Key points

- Luxatio erecta is a rare form of glenohumeral dislocation and occurs due to a severe hyperabduction injury to the arm.
- The patient presents with the extremity in a 'salute' position.
- Almost all cases are associated with transient neurovascular compromise, which usually resolves after reduction.
- Patients should be admitted post-reduction to monitor their neurovascular status.

References

1. Davids JR, Talbott RD. Luxatio erecta humeri: a case report. *Clin Orthop Relat Res* 1990; 252: 144-9.

2. Mallon WJ, Bassett FH, 3rd, Goldner RD. Luxatio erecta. *J Orthop Trauma* 1990; 4(1): 19-24.

Case 7

Clinical presentation

A 68-year-old woman presents to the ER after falling onto her outstretched right hand when she tripped over the curb while walking. She has no other injuries.

Physical examination

On physical exam, she is holding her left arm close to her body with her right arm. There is swelling over the proximal humerus and she is reluctant to move her shoulder. Sensation is intact over the lateral arm. Distally, she has no neurovascular deficits.

Review the images below [Figures 18 and 19]. Describe your findings.

Questions

1. What is the diagnosis?

2. What is the mechanism of injury?

3. Which two radiographic views of the shoulder are most important to obtain?

4. Describe the Neer classification system.

5. How do four-part proximal humerus fractures differ from the rest?

6. What is the anatomic structure that is most likely to be injured in these injuries?

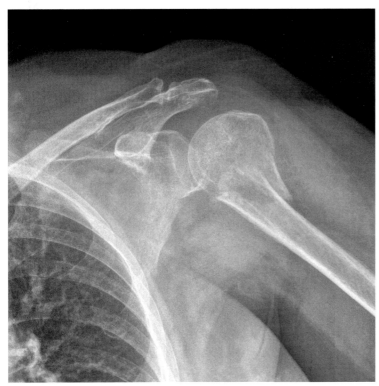

Figure 18.

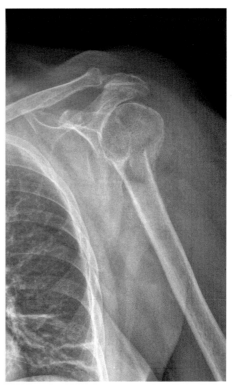

Figure 19.

Radiology findings

There is an oblique fracture through the surgical neck of the humerus. The distal fracture fragment is medially displaced. There is proximal impaction at the fracture site. A second fracture line is observed at the greater tuberosity, without displacement or angulation of fracture fragments.

Answers

1. Surgical neck fracture of the proximal humerus.

2. The mechanism of injury is axial loading on the outstretched extremity during a fall. These fractures are more commonly seen in older women as a result of osteoporosis. Proximal humeral fractures also occur in motor vehicle accidents with direct blows to the shoulder in a high-energy trauma.

3. AP and axillary views should be obtained. The injury is usually best characterized on the AP radiograph but the axillary view (or a modification that shows this axis) is essential to confirm that the humeral head is located in the glenoid (i.e. to rule out glenohumeral dislocation). Commonly, plain film views should be supplemented with a CT scan to fully assess the injury. Alternatively, a Velpeau axillary radiograph can be obtained (this is a reverse axillary view, where the patient is angled ~45° to the cassette and the X-ray is shot from above the shoulder).

4. The Neer system is the most commonly used classification system for proximal humerus fractures. Neer identified four bone fragments, referred to as parts:
   i)   the humeral head;
   ii) the humeral shaft;
   iii) the greater tuberosity; and
   iv) the lesser tuberosity.
   In this system, a part is defined as displaced only if there is either greater than 45° of angulation or greater than 1cm of fracture fragment displacement. This is often a point of confusion. A fracture can have multiple fragments; however, if none of these fragments are displaced, then the fracture is a one-part fracture. This is important, because these types of fractures are treated non-operatively. The Neer system can be further modified to include fracture-dislocation injuries and articular surface involvement:
   i)   one-part fractures have no or minimal displacement (less than 1cm or 45° of angulation), regardless of the number of fracture lines that may be present [Figure 20];
   ii) two-part fractures can involve any of the four parts, with one displaced fragment. They usually involve the humeral head or shaft, and not the tuberosities [Figure 21];
   iii) three-part fractures are two displaced fractures of both the surgical neck and either the greater or lesser tuberosities;
   iv) four-part fractures are injuries in which there is displacement of three segments, including both tuberosities [Figure 22].

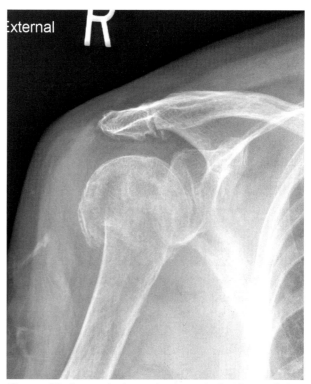

Figure 20. Impacted surgical neck fracture of the right humerus without displacement or angulation of fracture fragments, consistent with a Neer one-part injury.

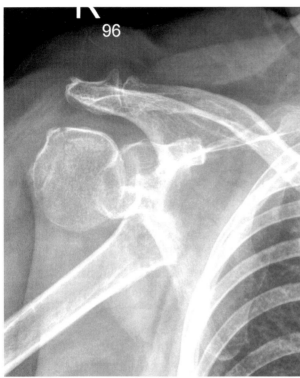

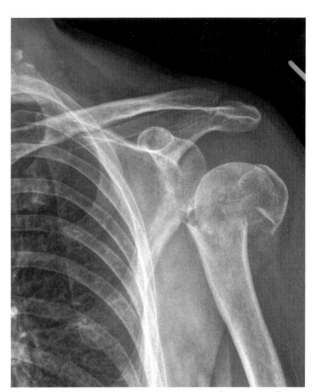

Figure 21. A fracture through the surgical neck of the humerus is present with marked antero-inferior displacement of the humeral shaft. The humeral head demonstrates additional fracture planes within but maintains its expected overall shape and remains within the glenoid fossa. This is consistent with a Neer two-part injury.

Figure 22. There is a comminuted fracture of the surgical neck of the humerus, with antero-inferior displacement of the distal fracture fragment. There is also a comminuted and displaced fracture of the greater tuberosity. There is pseudosubluxation of the humeral head secondary to a glenohumeral joint effusion. The lesser tuberosity is not clearly visualized and is likely displaced. Additional views are needed to confirm this. These findings are consistent with a four-part valgus impacted fracture of the humeral head, as classified by the Neer system. This injury is often underappreciated but the valgus impaction of the humeral head implies significant displacement and a poor prognosis.

5. A four-part proximal humerus fracture is the hardest type to treat as compared with the other Neer fracture types. There is a higher risk of osteonecrosis (avascular necrosis) of the humeral head due to the anatomical humeral neck fracture. The fracture fragments are small, unstable, and difficult to hold surgically. While surgical stabilization may be attempted, shoulder hemi-arthroplasty is also often performed. Patients are typically left with some degree of permanent stiffness and impaired function despite the method of treatment.

6. The structure most likely to be injured is the axillary nerve. This is most likely with anterior glenohumeral dislocations. The axillary nerve passes backwards under the inferior edge of the glenoid and exits through the quadrangular space. An anterior-inferior dislocation can stretch the nerve. Other potential complications include malunion, non-union, rotator cuff injuries, and shoulder stiffness. In the appropriate clinical setting (such as a motor vehicle accident), other co-injuries may be present such as chest trauma and associated fractures of the upper extremity.

Management

The fracture in this patient is managed conservatively. The patient is placed in a sling and swathe initially, and advised to use only a gentle range of motion, such as pendulums, starting approximately one week after the injury when the patient is more comfortable and swelling has decreased. This is done for stable fractures that are not likely to displace. The patient then progresses to a passive range of motion, and eventually an active range of motion as bony healing progresses.

Depending on the extent of the injury, the treatment will vary. For example, for the injuries pictured above, the treatment is as follows:

◆ Figure 20: this injury can be managed as the above example. It is essentially a non-displaced proximal humeral fracture.
◆ Figure 21: this displaced fracture is unstable and maintained there by strong local muscle forces. Initially a closed reduction may be attempted. The arm can be abducted and forced superiorly in an attempt to impact the fracture fragments. If this is successful, and the fracture remains stable, then the patient can be managed non-operatively with close follow-up. In this fracture, unopposed action of the pectoralis major and deltoid cause persistent displacement. Reduction may initially be successful but they rarely hold position and operative stabilization is usually required. An alternative is to place the patient in a collar and cuff sling to allow the effect of gravity to reduce the fragments. If there is good alignment, and minimal displacement, and the fracture remains stable over a period of 2-3 weeks, conservative management can be undertaken. If the conservative means fail, an open reduction with operative stabilization is required. In the frail elderly or with very high-energy fractures in younger patients, the marked medial displacement of the distal fragment may place the brachial plexus and axillary artery at risk.
◆ Figure 22: this is a four-part valgus impacted fracture. The best management is controversial with proponents for both non-operative and operative methods. With the latter, some surgeons prefer reconstruction and internal fixation while others will recommend hemi-arthroplasty.

The indications to operate on proximal humerus fractures are not black and white. Functional impairment and neurovascular structure compromise are factors to consider. If the fracture can be appropriately aligned by closed reduction, and function is acceptable for the patient, then non-surgical management will be successful.

Key points

◆ A complete shoulder series should be obtained of proximal humeral fractures to characterize the injury and to confirm that the shoulder is not dislocated. The axillary view is one of the most important views to obtain in these fractures but may be impossible in the painful acute trauma situation. A Velpeau axillary radiograph can also be obtained.
◆ The axillary nerve is the most likely structure to be injured.
◆ The goals of treatment are to obtain good functional outcome, and limit damage to neurovascular structures. If fractures are minimally displaced and stable, conservative management can be pursued.
◆ Management of more complex proximal humerus fractures is controversial, and requires specialist referral.

References

1. Neer CS, II. Displaced proximal humeral fractures. Part I. Classification and evaluation. *J Bone and Joint Surg* 1970; 52-A: 1079.
2. Koval KJ, Zuckerman JD. *Handbook of Fractures*, 3rd ed. Philadelphia, PA: Lippincott Williams & Wilkins, 2006.

Case 8

Clinical presentation

A 77-year-old woman presents to the ER after a fall onto her outstretched right hand. She did not hit her head, and did not lose consciousness. She is only complaining of right arm pain.

Physical examination

The patient is holding her right elbow with her left hand. There is swelling over the right arm. There is no gross deformity. When you gently move her arm, there is clear instability in the upper arm with crepitus. Distally, she has palpable radial and ulnar pulses, and good sensation in the radial nerve distribution. She can flex her elbow with pain, and can retropulse her thumb.

Review the images below [Figures 23 and 24]. Describe your findings.

Questions

1. What is the diagnosis?

2. What is the mechanism of injury?

3. On physical examination, what is the most important nerve to test?

4. Trace the course of this important nerve through the forearm.

5. How are most humeral shaft fractures managed? What are the indications for operative treatment for these types of injuries?

6. How are these injuries classified?

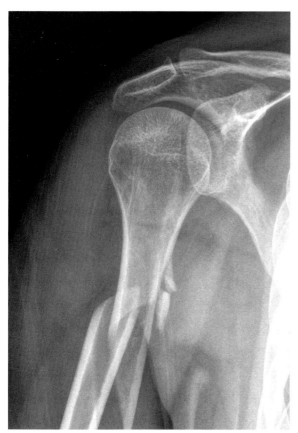

Figure 23.

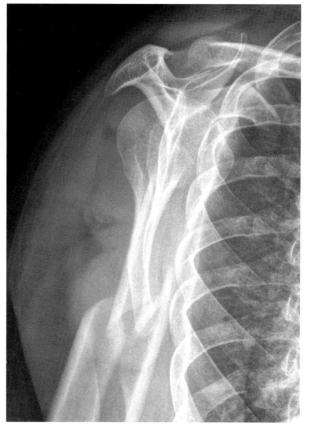

Figure 24.

Radiology findings

There is a spiral fracture of the proximal shaft of the humerus with posterior and superior displacement of the distal fracture fragment. The glenohumeral and AC joint spaces are well maintained.

Answers

1.   Spiral fracture of the proximal third of the humeral shaft.

2.   The mechanism of injury is a rotational force usually after a fall onto the arm. Specific mechanisms of injury produce specific fracture patterns. A direct force applied to the humeral shaft tends to produce a transverse fracture, with or without comminution and is likely to be seen after higher energy events. With more indirect forces, such as a fall onto an outstretched arm, the fracture is oblique or spiral. The latter happens as the patient axial loads the extremity, and in an attempt to break the fall the body twists about the arm as it is firmly planted on the ground, creating the rotational force. High-energy injuries are often seen in younger patients, and low-energy injuries are often seen in the elderly.

3.   Up to 20% of humerus shaft fractures are associated with radial nerve injury. This is most commonly seen with injuries at the junction of the middle and distal thirds of the humeral shaft, because the radial nerve lies closely applied to the bone in the spiral groove. A radial nerve palsy is usually due to a stretch injury and rarely an actual laceration. It commonly recovers and is not usually considered to be an indication for surgical treatment.

4.   The radial nerve is derived from the posterior cord of the brachial plexus. It passes through the quadrangular space, below the teres major muscle. It then runs between the medial and lateral heads of the triceps muscle in the spiral groove of the humerus. Above the elbow, it curves around the lateral epicondyle and exits between the brachialis and brachioradialis. Shortly after it exits, it splits into three branches:

one innervates the supinator and becomes the posterior interosseous nerve (PIN), one becomes the lateral cutaneous branch of the forearm, and the last continues distally underneath the brachioradialis with the radial artery. At the wrist, it exits above the abductor pollicis longus, courses over the extensor retinaculum, and provides sensation only to the dorsum of the hand.

5.   Most humeral shaft fractures are managed non-operatively. The indications for operative trauma include: a multi-trauma patient, where a fracture of the humerus will limit rehabilitation, pathological fractures, associated vascular injury, open fractures, intra-articular extension of the fracture, a 'floating elbow', malunion or non-union.

6.   In the Orthopedic Trauma Association/ Arbeitsgemeinschaft für Osteosynthesefragen (OTA/AO) system of fracture classification, the humerus is bone 1, the shaft zone is 2 and the specific fractures classified by the fracture pattern and degree of comminution are divided into A, B and C types. Sub-classifications can further detail the fracture into a number of more detailed subtypes. In common practice, simple descriptive terms are often used. It is important to describe whether the fracture is open or closed, its location (proximal, middle or distal third of the humeral shaft), displacement and angulation.

Management

Most humeral shaft fractures are managed non-operatively. A collar and cuff sling and coaptation splint (U slabs) will be applied initially to stabilize the limb for comfort. Use of gravity is an essential part of non-operative care with vertical posture and the weight of the arm often leading to good fracture reduction. The splint will usually be changed to a humeral brace after a short time and gentle pendulum exercises begun as soon as possible. The elbow should be allowed to extend intermittently as soon as possible. The patient will progress as comfort allows with more active exercises as possible. The splint can be discarded when the fracture is clinically stable and healing radiographically.

Key points

♦ Humeral shaft fractures can be associated with a radial nerve injury. The vast majority of simple radial nerve palsies in this situation recover spontaneously over several months.

♦ Oblique and spiral fractures are a sign of low-energy injury. Transverse and comminuted fractures are a sign of high-energy injury.

♦ 90% of humeral shaft fractures are treated non-operatively and heal well.

References

1. Thompson JC. *Netter's Concise Atlas of Orthopedic Anatomy.* Icon Learning Systems Inc., 2004.

2. Bucholz RW, Heckman JD, Court-Brown CM, *et al,* Eds. *Rockwood and Green's Fractures in Adults,* 6th ed. Philadelphia, PA: Lippincott Williams & Wilkins, 2006.

3. Koval KJ, Zuckerman JD. *Handbook of Fractures,* 3rd ed. Philadelphia, PA: Lippincott Williams & Wilkins, 2006.

Chapter 3

Elbow and distal humerus

Case 1

Clinical presentation

An 82-year-old woman slips and falls onto her bathroom floor. She lands on her left arm. She does not hit her head and does not lose consciousness. She presents to the ER with significant pain and swelling in her left elbow.

Physical examination

The skin is closed. There is significant swelling and ecchymosis of the left elbow. The patient holds the elbow flexed, close to her body. Range of motion is not possible secondary to pain. Distally, the patient has palpable radial and ulnar pulses, but reports decreased sensation over the palmar surface of her left thumb.

Review the images below [Figures 1 and 2]. Describe your findings.

Questions

1. What is the diagnosis?

2. What is the mechanism of injury?

3. Describe the columnar anatomy of the elbow. Why is this important?

4. What is the AO/OTA classification for these fractures?

5. What are some associated complications?

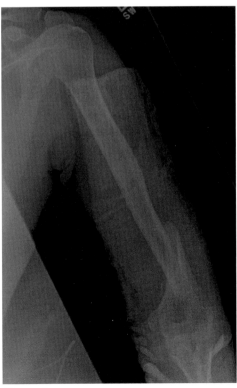

Figure 1.

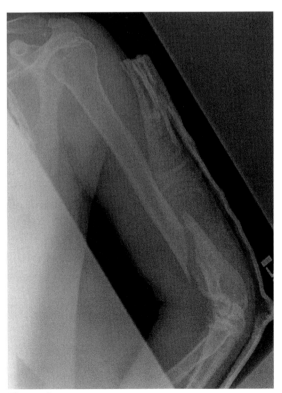

Figure 2.

Radiology findings

There is an oblique fracture of the left distal humeral shaft. The distal fragment is displaced posteriorly and with varus angulation compared with the proximal fragment. The fracture does not appear to extend into the joint line.

Answers

1. Oblique left distal humeral shaft fracture.

2. These injuries usually result from an axial load onto an outstretched hand, such as during a fall. Energy is transmitted from the proximal radius and ulna to the capitellum and trochlea, which contact the distal humerus and transmit the force causing the fracture.

3. The elbow is made up of a medial and lateral column. Each column is triangular in cross-section and has its respective condyles and epicondyles. The condyles are articulating, and the epicondyles are non-articulating. The forearm flexors originate at the medial epicondyle, and the forearm extensors originate at the lateral epicondyle. The medial column is composed of the medial epicondyle and medial condyle, and the medial humeral shaft. The lateral column is composed of the capitellum, lateral condyle, lateral epicondyle, and lateral humeral shaft. The trochlea lies in the middle and forms a tie arch between the distal part of each column. The articular surface is composed of the capitellum (lateral column), trochlea (tie arch), and medial condyle (medial column). Knowing the columnar anatomy of the elbow helps identify fracture fragments, classify/describe the fracture, and in a comminuted fracture, it can aid in reduction as each column is individually reconstructed and brought together.

4. The AO/ATO classification divides these fractures into three types:
    i) Type A: extra-articular fractures, and include epicondylar fractures, supracondylar fractures, and supracondylar fractures with comminution;
    ii) Type B: unicondylar fractures, such as fractures of the medial condyle, lateral condyle, or tangentially across the condyle;
    iii) Type C: bicondylar fractures, such as T-shaped or Y-shaped fractures involving both columns, with comminution, and with comminution involving the columns and condyles.

5. Complications include radial nerve injury, Volkmann's ischemic contracture (which may result from an unrecognized compartment syndrome), stiffness of the elbow after reconstruction, and heterotopic bone formation.

Management

The management of extra-articular distal humeral fractures is controversial, with proponents for operative and non-operative management. The approach used for the range of fractures will be determined by the amount of exposure needed to provide adequate reduction and stabilization of the individual fracture. Isolated lateral and medial condyle fractures can be treated with a Kocher approach and medial approach to the elbow, respectively, while more extensive fractures will require a greater exposure even with an olecranon osteotomy to allow full reflection of the triceps.

In general, plating techniques are utilized with as long a plate as possible for stability. In the extreme situation of a very low destructive fracture in elderly frail bone, an elbow arthroplasty may be considered.

Postoperatively, depending on the stability of fixation, range of motion of the elbow joint is started as soon as possible.

Key points

- Distal humerus fractures are best understood by visualizing the three columns of the elbow.

- The medial column is made up of the medial condyle and epicondyle. The lateral column is made up of the lateral condyle and capitellum.

- Options for reconstruction include plate fixation and screw fixation for healthy bone, versus considering a total elbow arthroplasty in poor quality bone with a comminuted fracture.

- Working around the triceps is the key to surgical exposure with both the ulna and radial nerves being at risk.

References

1.   Anglen J. Distal humerus fractures: surgical techniques. *J Am Acad Orthop Surg* 2005; 13: 291-7.

Case 2

Clinical presentation

A 22-year-old male is in a wrestling competition and while tackling his opponent, he falls landing on his left outstretched hand. He immediately notes pain and deformity of his left elbow, and presents to the ER for further evaluation.

Physical examination

On physical exam, there is gross deformity of the left elbow. There is swelling mostly posteriorly over the olecranon. The skin is intact. The patient guards the elbow close to his body and resists any examination of range of motion. Distally, he can flex and extend his wrist, spread apart his fingers, make an OK sign, and retropulse his thumb. He has palpable radial and ulnar pulses.

Review the images below [Figures 3 and 4]. Describe your findings.

Questions

1. What is the diagnosis?

2. What is the mechanism of injury?

3. What other injuries should you look for?

4. How are these injuries classified?

5. What long-term complications may occur?

6. In what direction does capsular and ligamentous injury occur?

7. What are the three articulations that make up the elbow joint?

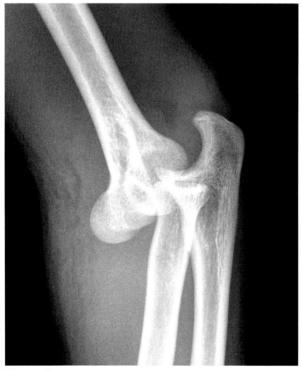

Figure 3.

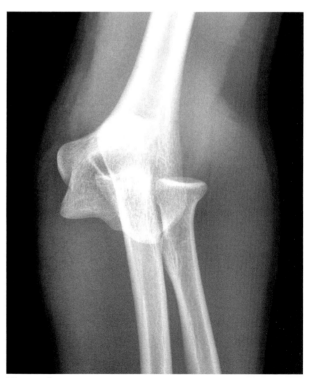

Figure 4.

Radiology findings

There is posterolateral dislocation of the elbow, or of the proximal ulna with respect to the distal humerus. There are no associated fractures.

Answers

1. Simple posterolateral elbow dislocation.

2. The mechanism of injury is a fall onto an outstretched hand. There is hyperextension of the elbow, valgus stress, forearm supination with the radius and ulna turning away from the humerus, and abduction of the arm, resulting in a posterolateral dislocation.

3. Associated injuries include damage to the surrounding joint capsule and ligaments. This may be evident if the joint is unstable after reduction. Posterior dislocations with an associated coronoid process and radial head fractures are known as terrible triad injuries.

4. Elbow dislocations are classified according to the direction of displacement of the proximal ulna relative to the distal humerus. There are six main directions: anterior, medial, lateral, posterior, posterolateral and posteromedial.

5. Simple, closed elbow dislocations are often reduced without subsequent complications. Rarely, there may be instability at the elbow joint. A small subset of patients may experience persistent subluxation and dislocation.

6. Injury to the capsular and ligamentous support of the elbow joint occurs in a lateral to medial fashion. The anterior band of the medial collateral ligament is the most important stabilizer to valgus stress of the elbow, and this is often uninjured in an elbow dislocation.

7. The three articulations are: proximal radio-ulnar, ulno-humeral, and radio-humeral.

Management

This dislocation can be reduced in the ER. The patient should be consciously sedated. For a posterior-lateral dislocation, longitudinal traction is applied with the elbow flexed at approximately 30-45°. One hand is placed on the humerus, and one on the midshaft radius and ulna. This will help unlock the distal ulna from the olecranon. First, medial/lateral deviation is corrected. While holding the elbow flexed at 45°, traction should continue to be applied, and the laterally displaced radial head should be pushed medially using the thumb and index finger of the hand holding onto the humerus. Now the posterior displacement can be corrected. The elbow is still flexed, traction is still applied, and with the hand holding the humerus, the olecranon is pushed anteriorly. The elbow should locate with a satisfying 'clunk.' In the pediatric population, performing the reduction independently is often possible because the upper extremity is small, and easily manipulated. In a more muscular adult, an assistant may be necessary to hold traction.

Once the joint is reduced, range of motion should be rechecked by flexing and extending the elbow. If it re-dislocates, the angle at which the dislocation occurs is noted. This is an unstable joint that will need operative fixation. If the joint does not re-dislocate, it is a stable injury. Also, after reduction, the neurovascular status of the limb should be re-evaluated.

The reduced elbow is placed in a posterior splint, flexed at 90°. If the joint was found to be unstable, the post-reduction films should be carefully reviewed for any associated fractures that may have been missed and an MRI may be obtained to evaluate the capsuloligamentous structures. If there is a stable reduction, gentle range of motion of the elbow can be started as soon as the patient is comfortable, and advanced as tolerated.

Key points

- The most common type of elbow dislocation is a posterior dislocation.

- A simple dislocation is one which is not associated with a fracture.

- After reduction, evaluation of the joint for stability is important.

- Associated fractures that may have been missed on the initial injury may be seen on post-reduction films, especially if the reduction is found to be unstable.

References

1. Cohen MS, Hastings H, 2nd. Acute elbow dislocation: evaluation and management. *J Am Acad Orthop Surg* 1998; 6(1): 15-23.

2. O'Driscoll SW. Elbow dislocations. In: *The Elbow and its Disorders*, 3rd ed. Morrey BF, Ed. Philadelphia, PA: WB Saunders, 2000: 409-17.

3. Rockwood CA Jr, Green DP, Bucholz RW, Eds. *Rockwood and Green's Fractures in Adults*, 4th ed. Philadelphia, PA: Lippincott Williams & Wilkins, 1996: 971-85.

Case 3

Clinical presentation

An 86-year-old female slips on the ice onto her outstretched arm, and presents with pain in her right elbow. She did not hit her head, and has no additional injuries.

Physical examination

On exam, the patient has a swollen right elbow, but the skin is intact. There is ecchymosis. She has pain when you attempt to range her elbow. Distally, she can make an OK sign, retropulse her thumb, and spread apart her fingers. She has no sensory deficits. She has palpable radial and ulnar pulses. She cannot extend her elbow with gravity eliminated.

Review the images below [Figures 5 and 6]. Describe your findings.

Questions

1. What is the diagnosis?

2. What is the mechanism of injury?

3. How are these injuries classified?

4. What complications may arise?

5. What is the primary indication for surgery?

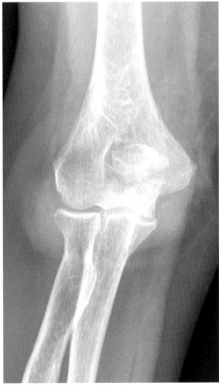

Figure 5.

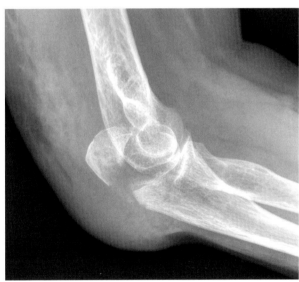

Figure 6.

Radiology findings

There is a transverse fracture through the olecranon with 11mm displacement of fracture fragments. The radial head is intact and there is no evidence of a dislocation.

Answers

1. Displaced fracture of the olecranon (Mayo Type II).

2. There are two main mechanisms that can result in olecranon fractures. The first is direct trauma to the elbow such as a fall. This causes comminution of the olecranon. The second is indirect trauma, such as a fall onto an outstretched extremity. This causes a transverse or oblique fracture of the olecranon.

3. The Mayo classification (Figure 7) is the most commonly used system to describe olecranon fractures and is based on displacement of fragments, comminution and ulnohumeral stability. There are three types of injuries according to this system:
   i) Type I: non-displaced or minimally displaced (<2mm) fractures which are either non-comminuted (Type IA) or comminuted (Type IB);
   ii) Type II: displaced proximal fragment without instability of the elbow, which are either non-comminuted (Type IIA) or comminuted (Type IIB);
   iii) Type III: fractures which are associated with ulnohumeral joint instability, and are either non-comminuted (Type IIIA) or comminuted (Type IIIB).

Mayo Type I
Undisplaced

Mayo Type II
Displaced
A - Non-comminuted
B - Comminuted

Mayo Type III
Accompanying lesions - instability
A - Non-comminuted
B - Comminuted

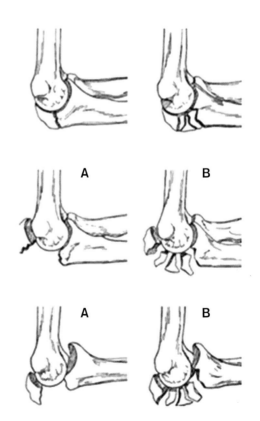

Figure 7. Mayo classification of olecranon fractures. *Reprinted with permission from Morrey BF, et al. The elbow and its disorders, 3d ed. Philadelphia: Saunders, 2000: 365-79. © Mayo Clinic Foundation, 2000.*

4. A fracture of the olecranon may be associated with an elbow dislocation or other fractures involving the radius, ulna, and humerus, and from injury to the ulnar nerve. Long-term complications include hardware failure, infection, heterotopic ossification, non-union, ulnar neuritis, and a decreased range of movement.

5. The main indication for surgery is incompetence of the extensor mechanism of the elbow. This should be tested with gravity eliminated. Softer indications include greater than 2mm of displacement, or incongruity of the articular surface at the elbow joint

Management

If the fracture is non-displaced/minimally displaced, and does not displace further when the arm is flexed to 90°, then it can be treated non-operatively in an elbow splint at 90° of flexion for 3-4 weeks. Then, active range of motion is started as tolerated.

For a displaced, simple fracture, a tension band is usually used. For a comminuted, displaced, unstable fracture, a dorsal plate with screws can provide adequate fixation.

In the case above, the patient was fixed using a dorsal plate with screws, as seen in the image below [Figure 8].

Key points

♦ The olecranon extends from the proximal ulna and articulates with the trochlea of the humerus.

♦ Olecranon fractures occur secondary to direct and indirect mechanisms and are grouped into three types according to the Mayo classification system.

♦ The ability to flex the elbow without further displacement of fracture fragments can help decide if surgery is indicated. Surgical options vary depending on the amount of comminution and displacement.

References

1. Bucholz RW, Heckman JD, Court-Brown CM, *et al*, Eds. *Rockwood and Green's Fractures in Adults*, 6th ed. Philadelphia, PA: Lippincott Williams & Wilkins, 2006.

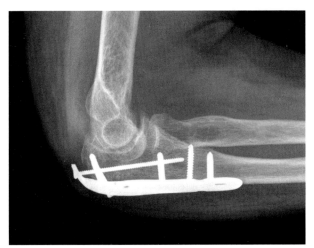

Figure 8. Post-ORIF of the olecranon fracture demonstrates satisfactory apposition of fracture fragments.

Case 4

Clinical presentation

A 29-year-old motorcyclist presents with severe left elbow pain after his bike skids off the road in a rainstorm. As the bike tipped onto its side, he was thrown off, landing onto his outstretched arm. He was wearing a helmet and had no loss of consciousness. He has severe road rash mostly over his left upper and lower extremities, and other than severe pain in his left elbow, is found to have no additional injuries.

Physical examination

On examination, there is obvious deformity of the left elbow with swelling and bruising both anteriorly and posteriorly. There are superficial abrasions, but no wounds likely to penetrate the deep layers. Any motion of his elbow is painful and resisted. Distally, there are no neurovascular deficits.

Review the images below [Figures 9 and 10]. Describe your findings.

Questions

1. What is the diagnosis?

2. What is the mechanism of injury?

3. What is the terrible triad?

4. What complications can arise?

5. What are the capsuloligamentous structures involved in elbow stability?

6. What nerve is at risk when repairing the coronoid process?

7. What nerve is at risk when working on the radial head?

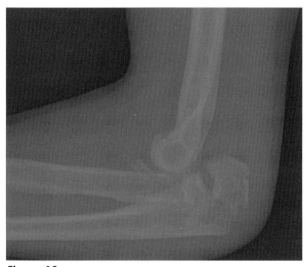

Figure 10.

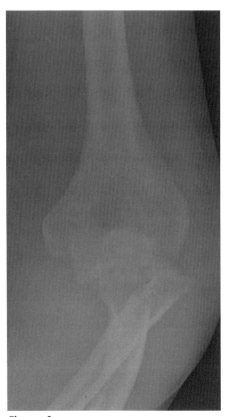

Figure 9.

Radiology findings

There is a posterior elbow dislocation, with an associated olecranon fracture, small fracture of the coronoid, and a fracture of the radial head.

Answers

1. Posterior elbow fracture-dislocation with an olecranon fracture and dislocation of the radial head.

2. As the elbow hyperextends, the olecranon is fractured and allows the elbow to dislocate posteriorly. The radial head and coronoid fracture as they contact the humerus during the dislocation. The lateral collateral ligament (LCL) is injured, followed by the medial collateral ligament (MCL).

3. When a coronoid fracture is associated with an elbow dislocation and a fracture of the radial head, this pattern is known as the 'terrible triad' (termed by Hotchkiss). This injury is important because there is increased elbow instability compared with other types of elbow dislocations (those without associated fractures or those only associated with a radial head fracture). There is also a higher incidence of complications.

4. Complications include joint stiffness, loss of motion, heterotopic ossification (myositis ossificans), ulnar neuropathy, non-union, malunion, infection, vascular compromise (most commonly involving disruption of the brachial artery), compartment syndrome (may require a forearm fasciotomy), proximal radio-ulnar synostosis and post-traumatic arthritis.

5. The MCL, LCL, and anterior capsule are involved in elbow stability. The MCL has an anterior, posterior, and transverse bundle. The anterior bundle is the most important stabilizer of the ligaments.

6. The ulnar nerve is held in place by Osbourne's fascia as it passes under the medial epicondyle.

When fixing the coronoid process, the ulnar nerve may need to be transposed.

7. The posterior interosseous nerve wraps around the radial neck. It is at risk of injury when a radial head resection or head replacement is performed.

Management

This is an unstable injury that will require operative fixation. The olecranon, radial head, and coronoid are fractured. The olecranon being a posterior structure, the coronoid a medial structure and the radial head a lateral structure, requires an approach to the elbow joint that will allow broad exposure posteriorly, medially, and laterally. A posterior triceps splitting approach to the elbow will most likely provide adequate exposure. Large tissue flaps can be raised through this approach. A contoured plate can be placed over the olecranon for fixation, the radial head can be replaced with a prosthesis, and the coronoid process can be repaired with sutures passed through the ulna by making drill holes. Alternatively, a screw can be placed through the ulna to hold the fractured coronoid in place. Once the bony anatomy is realigned, the LCL can be repaired. Usually the elbow heals well without the need to fix the MCL. So, if this ligament is torn, it can be left to heal on its own provided that the joint line bony anatomy is restored, and the LCL is repaired.

Often times it is difficult to determine exactly what structures are fractured in the elbow joint, especially to determine if the coronoid is fractured. If there is doubt, then a CT scan should be obtained to better identify the fractured elements.

Postoperatively, the patient is splinted at 90° of elbow flexion. Unlike with a simple elbow dislocation, initiation of range of motion begins at a slightly later time interval. The time for immobilization is usually between 1-3 weeks. After that gentle elbow range of motion is begun. The wrist can also become stiff after an elbow injury, and an appropriate physical therapy program should involve the ipsilateral wrist and elbow.

Key points

- The 'terrible triad' elbow fracture-dislocation includes a fracture of the radial head, fracture of the coronoid process, and an elbow dislocation.

- These injuries may require capsuloligamentous reconstruction, internal fixation, prosthetic replacement of the radial head, and/or external fixation.

- This is an unstable injury, and is usually treated operatively.

- Closed reduction in the ER should be attempted, despite the additional fractures, and the patient should be monitored closely for any signs of compartment syndrome if there is significant swelling.

References

1. Hotchkiss RN. Fractures of the radial head and related instability and contracture of the forearm. *Instr Course Lect* 1998; 47: 173-7.

2. Hotchkiss RN, Weiland AJ. Valgus stability of the elbow. *J Orthop Res* 1987; 5(3): 372-7.

3. Hotchkiss R. Fractures and dislocations of the elbow. In: *Fractures in Adults*. Rockwood CA, Green DP, Eds. Philadelphia, PA: Lippincott-Raven; 1996: 929-1024.

Case 5

Clinical presentation

A 63-year-old woman trips on a curb and falls onto her left outstretched arm. She presents to the ER complaining of pain in her elbow.

Physical examination

The skin over the elbow is intact, and there are no abrasions. There is mild swelling over the lateral elbow, but otherwise no gross deformity. The patient's flexion and extension of the elbow, as well as supination and pronation, are limited by pain. The distal radio-ulnar joint (DRUJ) is stable. The patient has no pain in her anatomic snuff box. There is also no pain or deformity of the humeral shaft.

Review the image below [Figure 11]. Describe your findings.

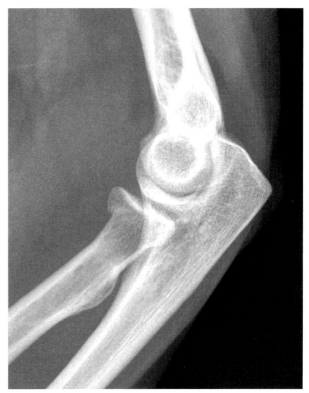

Figure 11.

Questions

1. What is the diagnosis?

2. What is the mechanism of injury?

3. How are these injuries classified?

4. What is the Essex-Lopresti lesion?

5. What other injuries might be present?

6. What is the 'safe zone' of the radial head?

Radiology findings

There is a minimally displaced (<2mm) fracture of the radial head with the presence of a posterior fat pad sign, indicating a joint effusion. When examining radiographs for a radial head fracture, search for the anterior sail sign or the posterior fat pad sign (more sensitive). These signs indicate a joint effusion and in the setting of trauma, this is strongly suggestive of a fracture of the radial head or neck. Often, the fracture line is not observed, but an occult fracture should be considered, especially in cases of positive physical examination findings. No other fractures are identified.

Answers

1. Non-displaced radial head fracture.

2. A fall onto an outstretched hand, causing axial loading of the radial head and fracture as it impacts against the capitellum.

3. This is a Mason Type I radial head fracture. Mason's classification system is most frequently used to categorize fractures of the radial head:
    i)   Type I injuries are non-displaced or minimally displaced (<2mm) fractures of the radial head or neck [Figure 12];
    ii) Type II injuries are displaced fractures of the radial head or neck (>2mm). There may be angulation, depression or impaction of fracture fragments;
    iii) Type III injuries are comminuted fractures of the radial head and neck. These injuries are not reconstructible. Type IV injuries include those radial head/neck fractures which are associated with dislocation of the elbow [Figure 13].

4. The Essex-Lopresti lesion is a disruption of the interosseous membrane of the forearm combined with a radial head fracture and/or dislocation, resulting in instability and subluxation of the DRUJ. This injury is often

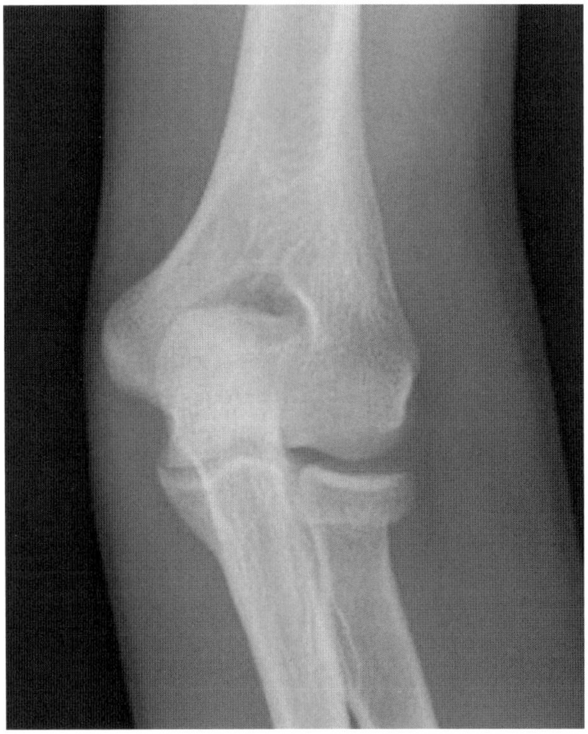

Figure 12. There is a transverse fracture of the radial neck with impaction at the fracture site. There is no significant angulation or displacement of fracture fragments. This is consistent with a Mason Type I injury.

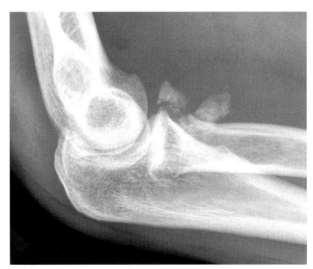

Figure 13. Comminuted fracture of the radial head seen after a reduction of an associated elbow dislocation.

missed because it is difficult to diagnose. If a patient is complaining of wrist pain with an associated radial head fracture, an Essex-Lopresti lesion is a possibility. The reason this injury is important is because it affects treatment. With a torn interosseous membrane, removal of the radial head can cause proximal migration of the radius. Therefore, the radial head should either be repaired or replaced with a prosthetic component to maintain radial length and the appropriate relationship between the two forearm bones.

5. Associated injuries include fracture of the capitellum (although this is rare). Other fractures include those that are caused by a similar mechanism, such as those of the distal radius, proximal ulna, lateral humeral condyle, olecranon, coronoid process, scaphoid, or humeral shaft. Patients may present with rupture of the MCL or an associated elbow dislocation. The terrible triad is a very unstable elbow injury involving a radial head fracture associated with a coronoid process fracture and MCL rupture. This is difficult to treat and has a high incidence of complications.

6. The safe zone of the radial head is the portion that does not articulate with the ulna. When looking at the radius in the anatomic position, with the arm in supination, the safe zone is the posterior-lateral quadrant of the radial head. This is important because it is the area of the radial head where plate or screw fixation can be placed, without interfering with the articulation of the proximal radio-ulnar joint.

Management

This relatively non-displaced fracture can be treated non-operatively, with the affected extremity in a sling, and range of motion of the elbow can begin as soon as the patient is comfortable. Aspiration of the hematoma under sterile conditions may significantly improve the acute discomfort by decompressing the elbow joint effusion.

Operative indications include:

♦   If there is a displaced radial head fracture that is causing a mechanical block to motion and cannot be closed reduced.
♦   Fracture of the radial head combined with a more complex elbow/arm injury, such as in a Monteggia fracture.
♦   Fractures of the radial head combined with elbow dislocation.

Key points

♦   Occult fractures of the radial head and neck are suggested by the presence of an elbow effusion (indicated by the anterior sail sign and/or posterior fat pad sign).
♦   Most radial head fractures can be managed non-operatively.
♦   The safe zone of the radial head is the posterior-lateral quadrant with the radius supinated and in anatomic position. The radial head contributes to valgus stability of the elbow.
♦   Remember to examine the DRUJ to assess for instability.

References

1. Mason ML. Some observations on fractures of the head of the radius with a review of one hundred cases. *Br J Surg* 1954; 42: 123-32.
2. Koval KJ, Zuckerman JD. *Handbook of Fractures*, 3rd ed. Philadelphia, PA: Lippincott Williams & Wilkins, 2006.

Case 6

Clinical presentation

A 63-year-old woman presents to the ER with pain and swelling in her elbow after a fall onto an outstretched hand.

Physical examination

On exam there is swelling of the patient's right elbow. The skin is intact. She has limited flexion and pain with supination and pronation. There are no neurovascular deficits.

Review the images below [Figures 14 and 15]. Describe your findings.

Questions

1. What is the diagnosis?

2. What is the mechanism of injury?

3. How are these injuries classified?

4. What complications can occur?

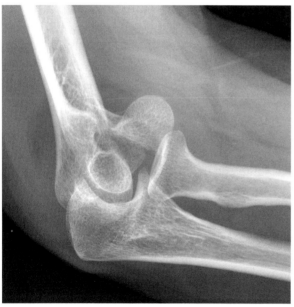

Figure 14.

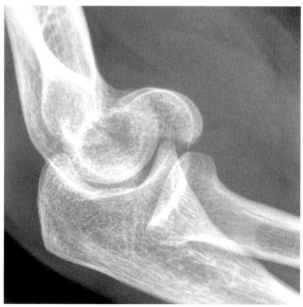

Figure 15.

Radiology findings

There is a complete fracture of the osseous part of the capitellum. It is significantly displaced. No other fractures are identified and there is no elbow dislocation.

Answers

1. Fracture of the capitellum.

2. A fall onto an outstretched hand, with axial loading of the extremity and transmission of the force from the radial head to the capitellum, is the most common mechanism.

3. These fractures are divided into two groups. In Type I injuries, there is a Hahn-Steinthal fragment which is a fracture of a large osseous part of the capitellum. In Type II injuries, there is a Kocher-Lorenz fragment, which is articular cartilage with minimal attached subchondral bone. The other classification system that is used is the Bryan and Morrey system. It is divided into three types:
   i) Type I: complete osteochondral fracture;
   ii) Type II: superficial osteochondral fracture fragment;
   iii) Type III: comminuted fracture.

4. Complications which may occur include post-traumatic osteoarthritis, stiffness, and osteonecrosis of the capitellar fragment.

Management

Those fractures that are non-displaced can be treated in a posterior splint for approximately three weeks, followed by range of motion of the elbow. If these fractures involve displacement of a major intra-articular fragment, they need surgical reduction and stabilization to restore the anatomy and stability of the articular surface. Type I fractures are usually treated through a posterolateral approach to the elbow, with a screw placed postero-anteriorly to hold the reduced capitellum. With Type II fractures, since there is little subchondral bone on the displaced capitellar fragment, they may not be reconstructible and may need treatment with excision of the fragment. Assuming stable fixation is obtained operatively, range of motion should begin as soon as the patient is comfortable.

Key points

- Axial loading by a fall onto an outstretched hand is a common mechanism of injury.
- Type I fractures can be treated by screw fixation; Type II fractures, due to the limited subchondral bone of the displaced fragments, are usually treated by excision.
- On exam, limited flexion, as well as pain with limited supination and pronation, indicate pathology in the joint.

References

1. Bryan RS, Morrey BF. Fractures of the distal humerus. In: *The Elbow and its Disorders*. Morrey BF, Ed. Philadelphia, PA: WB Saunders, 1985: 302-39

2. Bucholz RW, Heckman JD, Court-Brown CM, *et al*, Eds. *Rockwood and Green's Fractures in Adults*, 6th ed. Philadelphia, PA: Lippincott Williams & Wilkins, 2006.

Case 7

Clinical presentation

A 42-year-old woman presents to the ER after a fall onto her left outstretched hand two days prior. Her left elbow is painful, especially with any range of motion. She has been icing and resting her left arm, but the pain is not improving.

Physical examination

On examination, she has some swelling over the posterior aspect of her elbow. The skin is intact, and there is no bruising. The elbow can be flexed and extended from just under 90° to 10° of extension. She has pain and limited pronation and supination, but the elbow does not feel unstable. Distally, she has no neurovascular deficits.

Review the image below [Figure 16]. Describe your findings.

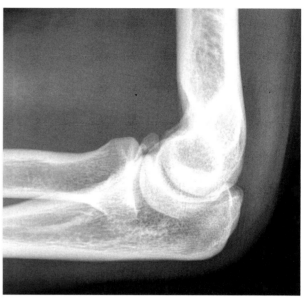

Figure 16.

Questions

1. What is the diagnosis?

2. What is the mechanism of injury?

3. How are these injuries classified?

4. List some complications that may occur.

Radiology findings

There is a mildly displaced fracture of the tip of the coronoid process. There is no associated elbow dislocation or fracture of the radial head. There is a posterior fat pad sign, indicating a joint effusion.

Answers

1. Avulsion fracture of the coronoid process (Type IA).

2. These injuries usually occur during axial loading after a fall onto an outstretched hand.

3. Fractures of the coronoid process are divided into three groups:
   i) Type I injuries are avulsion fractures of the tip of the coronoid process;
   ii) Type II injuries consist of a single or comminuted fracture fragment involving less than 50% of the coronoid process;
   iii) Type III injuries consist of a single or comminuted fracture fragment involving greater than 50% of the coronoid process.
   Each injury is further sub-classified into A (isolated fractures) and B (those associated with an elbow dislocation). The most severe is the associated injuries of the terrible triad, consisting of an elbow dislocation, radial head fracture and coronoid process fracture.

4. Complications include elbow instability or stiffness and post-traumatic osteoarthritis or heterotopic ossification. In Type II and III injuries, patients may suffer from nerve damage involving the ulnar, median, radial and anterior interosseous nerves. The brachial artery is rarely involved in isolated fractures.

Management

A Type I fracture, with a stable elbow as in the patient above, can be treated with conservative management using a sling, a long arm posterior splint, and limited use of the affected extremity for approximately three weeks. After this, point range of motion is begun, and the patient is slowly progressed to full weight bearing of the affected extremity. A minimally displaced Type II fracture can also be treated in a similar fashion. For a Type III injury, displaced Type II, or those associated with an elbow dislocation, the stability of the elbow is the key factor determining treatment. If an elbow dislocation is present, it should be reduced in the ER, and the patient placed in a posterior splint. Stability of the elbow should be determined. If the elbow is unstable, surgery for definitive fixation using open reduction with internal fixation (ORIF) is recommended. The terrible triad combination injury requires reconstruction of all three elements of the injury.

Key points

◆ Most Type II and III injuries require operative fixation.

◆ The main determinant of surgical versus conservative management is based on the stability of the elbow.

◆ The terrible triad is an elbow dislocation associated with a radial head fracture and coronoid process fracture. These are unstable injuries.

References

1. Regan W, Morrey B. Fractures of the coronoid process of the ulna. *J Bone Joint Surg* 1989; 71A: 1348-54.

2. Selesnick FH, Dolitsky D, Haskell SS. Fracture of the coronoid process requiring open reduction with internal fixation. *J Bone Joint Surg* 1984; 66A: 1304-5.

3. Bucholz RW, Heckman JD, Court-Brown CM, *et al*, Eds. *Rockwood and Green's Fractures in Adults*, 6th ed. Philadelphia, PA: Lippincott Williams & Wilkins, 2006.

Chapter 4

Wrist and forearm

Case 1

Clinical presentation

An 18-year-old man is brought into the ER by his peers. A group of young men were in a brawl, and the patient was struck on the thigh and shoulder with a bat. He threw his left arm up to protect his head and the bat struck his left arm. He is found to have the injury seen below.

Physical examination

The patient has swelling over the mid-ulnar border of his left arm. There is redness and bruising over the area where the bat struck. The skin is intact. The patient is tender to palpation, and crepitus is felt over the midshaft of the ulna. Distally, he has only minor pain with wrist range of motion. Proximally, he has only minor pain with elbow range of motion. He has no neurovascular deficits.

Review the images below [Figures 1 and 2]. Describe your findings.

Questions

1. What is the diagnosis?

2. What is the mechanism of injury?

3. What are the possible complications?

4. What factors help determine whether this injury is unstable?

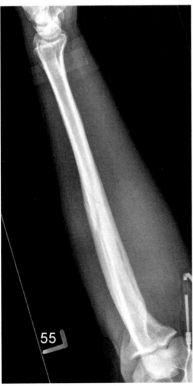

Figure 1.

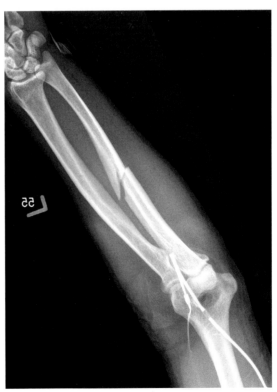

Figure 2.

Radiology findings

There is an oblique fracture of the midshaft of the left ulna with a 3mm radial displacement of the distal fracture segment. There is no significant angulation at the fracture site. There is no evidence of a radial head dislocation.

Answers

1. Isolated ulnar shaft fracture.

2. Ulnar shaft fractures most commonly occur secondary to a direct blow to the forearm. Historically, they are also known as a nightstick fracture, occurring after a victim tries to protect themselves from an injury by raising their arm in front of them. These fractures are also associated with motor vehicle accidents and other high-energy trauma. Although not as common, an isolated ulnar shaft fracture may result from a fall from height.

3. Non-union is a potential complication which is seen in approximately 5% of cases. Studies have found that the risk for non-union is due to a multitude of factors, including proximal fracture site, displacement of fragments, comminution and early mobilization. Other complications that may occur after an isolated ulnar shaft fracture include radio-ulnar synostosis, and loss of motion.

4. Unstable ulnar shaft fractures include those that are displaced more than 50%, angulated more than 10-15°, or are located in the proximal third of the ulna. The periosteum and interosseous membranes are disrupted and there may be associated injuries (radial head fracture or dislocation).

Management

Fractures that are displaced less than one half a shaft's width and that are angulated less than 10° can be treated with immobilization in a short arm cast. Those fractures that are displaced greater than one

half a shaft, or have significant angulation can be treated surgically with open reduction and internal fixation (ORIF) using a compression plate. In the patient above, there appears to be minimal displacement of the fracture in the lateral plane, minimal angulation, and less than one half a shaft's width translation in the AP plane. This patient can be treated non-operatively. However, the angulation in this fracture is directed towards the interosseous membrane as seen on the AP view and there may be some rotation at the fracture site. This is often uncomfortable for patients and can be a sign of instability. It is not unreasonable to offer this patient surgical fixation.

Key points

♦ Isolated ulnar shaft fractures are common and are typically seen after a direct blow to the forearm.

♦ Unstable injuries are those that are angulated more than 10-15°, displaced more than 50%, are located in the proximal ulna, or are displaced towards the interosseous membrane.

♦ Management options for stable injuries include immobilization in a sugar-tongue splint or a short arm cast. For unstable injuries, these can be treated with ORIF using a compression plate as one means of fixation.

References

1. Goel SC, Raj KB, Srivastava TP. Isolated fractures of the ulnar shaft. *Injury* 1991; 22(3): 212-4.

2. Brakenbury PH, Corea JR, Blakemore ME. Non-union of the isolated fracture of the ulnar shaft in adults. *Injury* 1981; 12(5): 371-5.

3. Sauder DJ, Athwal GS. Management of isolated ulnar shaft fractures. *Hand Clin* 2007; 23(2): 179-84, vi.

Case 2

Clinical presentation

A 32-year-old obese woman presents to the ER after falling onto her right outstretched hand.

Physical examination

There is swelling over the distal forearm including the wrist. There is a deformity at the wrist. The skin is intact. The patient has pain on palpation over the distal forearm, and has an unstable distal radio-ulnar joint (DRUJ). She has palpable radial and ulnar pulses, and sensation is intact in the radial, median, and ulnar nerve distribution. She has no motor deficits in her hand, although she hesitates to move her thumb and fingers secondary to pain.

Review the images below [Figures 3 and 4]. Describe your findings.

Questions

1. What is the diagnosis?

2. What is the mechanism of injury?

3. Why is this fracture often referred to as a 'fracture of necessity?'

4. How are these injuries classified?

5. What are some of the complications that can occur?

6. What are the four important signs to identify on a radiograph that indicate disruption of the DRUJ?

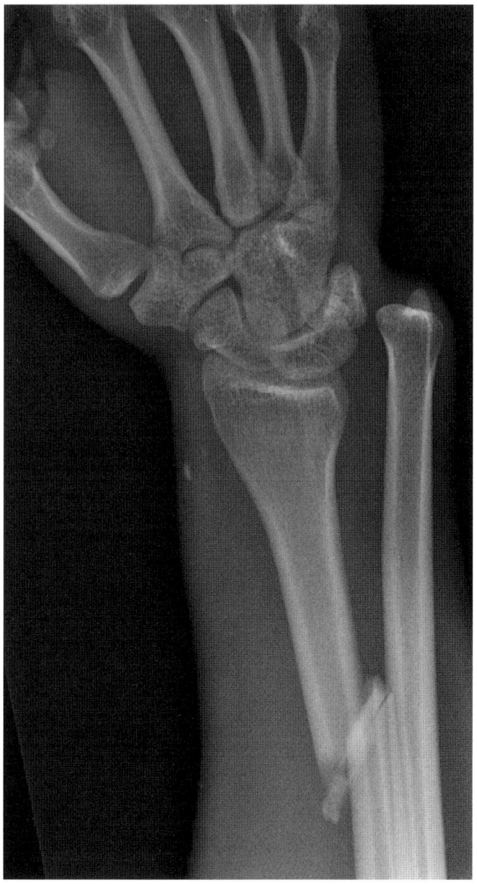

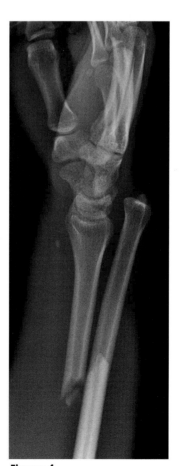

Figure 3.

Figure 4.

Radiology findings

There is an oblique fracture of the radial shaft at the junction of the middle and distal thirds with volar displacement at the fracture site. The distal ulna lies dorsal to the displaced distal radius with a dislocation of the DRUJ.

Answers

1. Galeazzi fracture (fracture of the radius with dislocation of the distal radio-ulnar joint [Figure 5]).

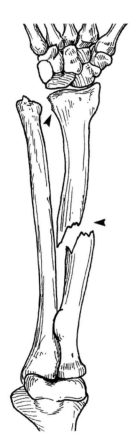

Figure 5. Depiction of a Galeazzi fracture. *Reprinted with permission from the Radiological Society of North America. Hunter T, Peltier L, Lund P, et al. Musculoskeletal eponyms: who are those guys? Radiographics 2000; 20(3): 819-36.*

2. These injuries typically result from a fall onto the outstretched hand with the elbow in a flexed

position (the forearm is pronated). They can also be seen after a direct blow to the dorsolateral aspect of the wrist.

3. This is called a 'fracture of necessity' because the only way to obtain adequate reduction is through operative means. The fracture loses reduction without internal fixation because:
    i)   the weight of the hand causes dorsal angulation of the radial shaft fracture with resultant disruption of the DRUJ;
    ii) the pronator quadratus originates on the medial distal ulna, and inserts on the anterior distal radius. The insertion site pronates the distal radial fragment;
    iii) the brachioradialis originates from the lateral supracondylar humerus, and attaches onto the lateral distal radius. The attachment site causes shortening.
    In order to restore the DRUJ, the radius needs to be anatomically reduced and surgically stabilized in the anatomical position. The thumb abductors (abductor pollicis brevis, flexor pollicis brevis, and opponens pollicis), as well as the extensor pollicis longus and brevis, pull on the radial collateral ligament, which prevents ulnar reduction from being maintained.

4. This is a Walsh Type II injury. Galeazzi fractures can be classified according to the position of the radius, known as the Walsh classification. In Type I injuries, there is dorsal displacement of the distal radius, whereas in Type II injuries, there is volar displacement of the distal radius.

5. In unstable injuries, there is a high incidence of non-union, delayed union and malunion. Other complications which can occur include neurovascular injury, usually iatrogenic, involving the superficial radial nerve. This nerve is located under the brachioradialis and is damaged with the Henry approach which uses the interval between the flexor carpi radialis and brachioradialis. Compartment syndrome is another important complication to watch for. Radio-ulnar synostosis is a rare complication that may occur. Distal radio-ulnar instability or even repetitive episodes of true dislocation are additional risks.

6. Injury to the DRUJ can be reliably identified on radiographs by observing four possible signs. These include:
   i) a fracture of the base of the ulnar styloid;
   ii) widening of the DRUJ on an AP view;
   iii) greater than 5mm of radial shortening. If radial shortening exceeds 10mm, this suggests complete disruption of the interosseous membrane;
   iv) shortening and subluxation or dislocation of the radius relative to the ulna seen on a lateral view.

Management

This fracture should be treated operatively. The anterior approach to the distal radius (also known as the Henry approach) is usually used to obtain adequate exposure of the fracture and apply appropriate plate fixation. With reduction of the shaft fracture, the DRUJ should also reduce. If it requires additional stability, Kirshner wires can be placed through the joint. With plate fixation of the radius and a stable DRUJ, range of motion can begin as soon as the patient is comfortable. With plate fixation and an unstable DRUJ, the wrist may require longer-term immobilization with a delayed range of motion.

Key points

- A Galeazzi fracture is a radial fracture with associated dislocation of the DRUJ.
- It is called the fracture of necessity because adequate reduction is difficult to maintain without internal fixation due to the intrinsic fracture instability and need for an anatomic reduction. Multiple muscle groups act on the distal third of the radial shaft and cause fracture deformity.
- A Henry approach to the radius with a volar plate can be used to fix the fracture.
- Stability of the DRUJ can determine how early the patient begins range of motion postoperatively.

References

1. Koval KJ, Zuckerman JD. *Handbook of Fractures*, 3rd ed. Philadelphia, PA: Lippincott Williams & Wilkins, 2006: 222-5.
2. Thompson JC. *Netter's Concise Atlas of Orthopedic Anatomy.* Icon Learning Systems Inc., 2002: 106-8.
3. Walsh HPJ, McLaren CANP. Galeazzi fractures in children. *J Bone Joint Surg Br* 1987; 69: 730-3.

Case 3

Clinical presentation

A 20-year-old woman presents to the ER with left wrist pain. She has had this pain for the last two days. She reports that it began after she fell down rollerblading and injured her left wrist. She has been icing her wrist and resting it, but has found no relief.

Physical examination

On physical exam, there is swelling over the left ulnar styloid process. The skin is intact. The area is tender to palpation. The patient has pain with wrist flexion and extension. Her DRUJ is stable on stress testing. She has no neurovascular deficits.

Review the images below [Figures 6 and 7]. Describe your findings.

Questions

1. What is the diagnosis?

2. What is the mechanism of injury?

3. What other injuries may also be present?

4. What important complication may arise?

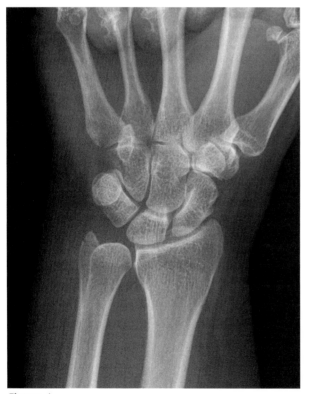

Figure 6.

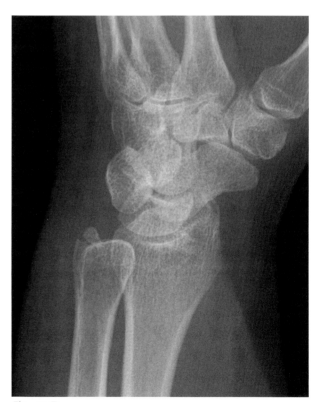

Figure 7.

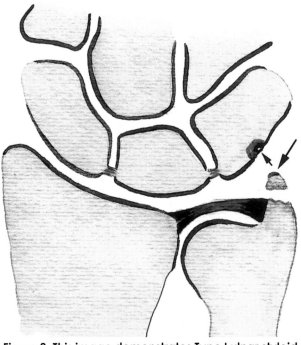

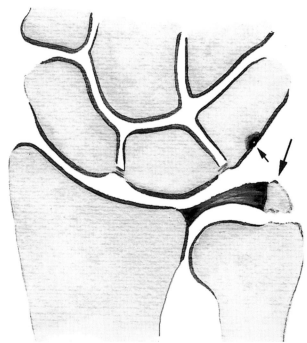

Figure 8. This image demonstrates Type I ulnar styloid non-union, with the TFCC and DRUJ intact. The non-united fragment acts as an irritant and results in focal chondromalacia of the triquetrum (short arrow) and subcortical sclerosis on the tip of the fragment (long arrow). *Reprinted with permission from the Radiological Society of North America. Cerezal L, del Piñal F, et al. Imaging findings in ulnar-sided wrist impaction syndromes. Radiographics 2002; 22(1): 105-21.*

Figure 9. This image demonstrates Type II ulnar styloid non-union, with avulsion of the TFCC cartilage, resulting in instability of the DRUJ. Also identified is focal chondromalacia and subcortical sclerosis. *Reprinted with permission from the Radiological Society of North America. Cerezal L, del Piñal F, et al. Imaging findings in ulnar-sided wrist impaction syndromes. Radiographics 2002; 22(1): 105-21.*

Radiology findings

There is a transverse fracture through the base of the ulnar styloid process, demonstrating minimal displacement of fracture fragments. No other fractures are identified. The distal radius is intact.

Answers

1. Isolated fracture of the ulnar styloid process.

2. Fractures of the ulnar styloid process typically occur after forced radial dorsiflexion.

3. The majority of ulnar styloid process fractures are associated with fractures of the distal radius (approximately 70-75%). There may also be an

associated injury to the triangular fibrocartilage complex (TFCC) resulting in disruption of the DRUJ. Fractures of the tip of the ulnar styloid process are usually accompanied with fractures of the distal radius and are of little clinical significance, as no major ligamentous structures tend to be affected. On the other hand, fractures at the base of the ulnar styloid process can be unstable due to involvement of the TFCC and hence the DRUJ. Instability is largely determined by clinical examination.

4. Non-union of the ulnar styloid process is an important but under-reported complication that may arise. Studies have described two types of non-union which may occur. The first, Type I, is non-union associated with a stable DRUJ [Figure 8]. This type affects fractures at the tip

of the ulnar styloid process, with an intact TFCC. The second, Type II, is non-union associated with subluxation of the DRUJ due to avulsion of the TFCC complex [Figure 9]. With both types of non-union, there may be impingement of the extensor carpi ulnaris tendon sheath, focal chondromalacia of the triquetrum and subcortical sclerosis of the non-united fragment. The patient may be asymptomatic, or experience pain and tenderness secondary to irritation and inflammation of the non-united segment.

Management

Most ulnar styloid fractures can be treated non-operatively by immobilizing the wrist, either in a removable type Charnley splint, or a short arm cast, for 4-6 weeks. Fixation of these fractures is controversial. If there is non-union of the ulnar styloid causing irritation in the wrist, and the TFCC is found to be intact (Type I non-union), then the fragment can simply be excised. If the DRUJ is unstable, and there is non-union of the ulnar styloid (Type II non-union), the fracture can be reduced with Kirschner wire percutaneous pinning of the fragment. The wrist is immobilized and monitored for healing.

Key points

♦ The most minimally displaced ulnar styloid fractures can be treated non-operatively.

♦ If the patient is found to have DRUJ instability and an ulnar styloid fracture, or a displaced ulnar styloid fracture, consideration is given to operative management.

♦ There are two types of non-union. In Type I, the apex of the styloid is fractured and the DRUJ is stable. In Type II, the fracture is at the base of the styloid and the DRUJ has the potential for instability.

References

1. Cerezal L, del Piñal F, *et al.* Imaging findings in ulnar-sided wrist impaction syndromes. *Radiographics* 2002; 22(1): 105-21.

2. Hauck RM, Skahen J, Palmer AK. Classification and treatment of ulnar styloid nonunion. *J Hand Surg [Am]* 1996; 21: 418-22.

3. Loftus JB, Palmer AK. Disorders of the distal radioulnar joint and triangular fibrocartilage complex: an overview. In: *The Wrist and its Disorders.* Lichtman DM, Alexander AH, Eds. Philadelphia, PA: Saunders, 1997: 385-414.

Case 4

Clinical presentation

A 62-year-old left-hand dominant woman presents to the ER after a mechanical fall on ice. She landed on her left outstretched hand. She has no additional injuries.

Physical examination

The left hand is grossly deformed, presenting as a dinnerfork appearance. There is diffuse swelling of the wrist, but the overlying skin is intact. Distally, the patient can make an OK sign, retropulse her thumb, and spread apart her fingers. She has palpable radial and ulnar pulses, and sensation is intact at the back of the hand, tips of the fingers, and over the small finger. Assessment of the DRUJ is impossible due to pain and swelling.

Review the images below [Figures 10 and 11]. Describe your findings.

Questions

1. What is the diagnosis?

2. What is the mechanism of injury?

3. What should you look for on plain films?

4. What finding would convince you to take the patient to the OR sooner rather than later?

5. List some important complications of these injuries.

6. What tendon is commonly injured?

7. What is the reverse pattern of this injury known as?

8. How are these injuries classified?

9. What are the normal measurements for distal radius length, inclination, and palmar tilt?

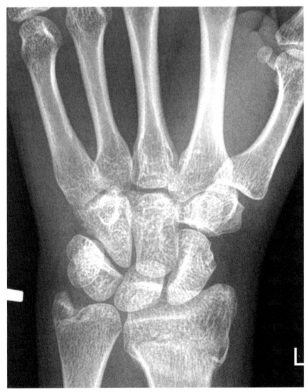

Figure 10.

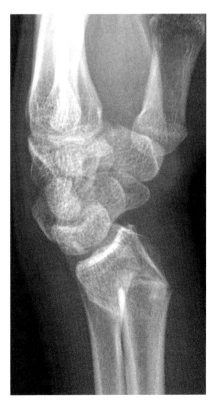

Figure 11.

Radiology findings

There is an impacted extra-articular fracture through the metaphyses of the distal radius. There is radial shortening (measuring 1.8cm) with a resultant ulnar deformity. The distal fragment is radially displaced and there is dorsal angulation of this fragment (measuring 37°). A transverse fracture through the base of the ulnar styloid process is also noted, and may suggest injury to the TFCC. Scapholunate dissociation is not identified, but there is disruption of the congruency of the DRUJ.

Answers

1. Dorsally displaced distal radius fracture (also known as a Colles' fracture).

2. The most common mechanism of injury is a fall on the outstretched hand. The forearm is typically pronated and the wrist is hyperextended and radially deviated.

3. When evaluating distal radial fractures, determination of stability is important as it predicts the likely success of non-operative treatment. Non-displaced fractures can be treated non-operatively but displaced and angulated fractures need manipulation and casting. Instability will produce a deformity after healing with significant radial shortening, deviation and dorsal displacement. Radiological findings to suggest instability include intra-articular involvement [Figure 12], dorsal angulation, an abnormal radial angle, palmar tilt, radial shortening/comminution, distal radio-ulnar subluxation and the presence of an associated ulnar styloid fracture.

4. Excruciating pain in a distal radial fracture is often a sign of impending carpal tunnel syndrome (CTS) with compression due to swelling/deformity on the median nerve. If a patient in the ER continues to have pain that is difficult to control, they should not be dismissed as having pain secondary to the fracture. The function of the median nerve should be re-

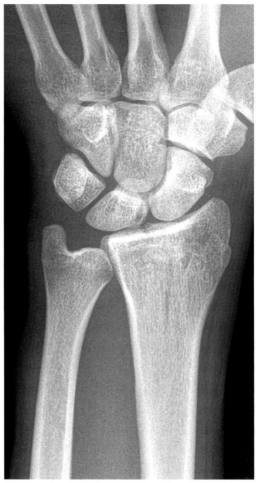

Figure 12. There is a comminuted fracture of the distal radius with the fracture lines primarily oriented in the vertical plane. There is extension into the articular surface. This is an impacted radial styloid fracture.

examined and reassessed. This may be a patient whose injury should be quickly reduced and if symptoms do not rapidly improve, they should be admitted and observed or taken to the operating theater for decompression.

5. Depending on the instability and associated ligamentous injury, complications vary and are divided into early and late. Early complications include median nerve dysfunction, acute carpal tunnel syndrome, compartment syndrome and tendon injury/rupture. Late complications include malunion or non-union, post-traumatic osteoarthritis, midcarpal instability, reflex

sympathetic dystrophy, wrist and hand stiffness, deformity, chronic DRUJ instability and tendon rupture.

6. The extensor pollicis longus tendon is the tendon most commonly injured. This is seen in both acute and chronic injuries. Even with adequate reduction and minimal displacement, the tendon may still be injured and may rupture late.

7. The opposite of a dorsally displaced fracture is a volarly displaced distal radial fracture. This is known as a Smith's fracture (or reverse Colles' fracture) [Figure 13]. These injuries result from a fall on an outstretched hand, with the hand in hyperflexion. Smith's fractures are classified according to the direction of the fracture line.

The 'garden spade deformity' results from volar (palmar) angulation of the distal radial fracture fragment. These fractures are often more difficult to closed reduce and if closed treatment is chosen, splintage is needed in supination.

8. Historically, there are a number of classification systems which have been proposed to classify fractures of the distal radius. However, the most important and useful classification system is the descriptive one. This best helps the orthopedic surgeon determine operative planning and overall morbidity of the injury. Injuries should initially be divided into intra and extra-articular. Other factors to take into account are dorsal or volar angulation, fracture fragment displacement, radial shortening, and involvement of the DRUJ.

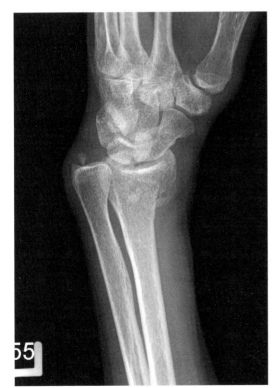 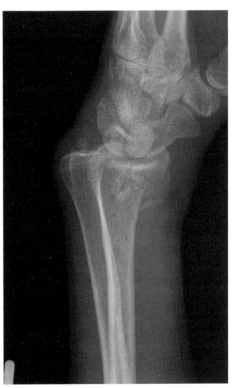

Figure 13. There is an oblique fracture of the distal radial metaphysis extending from the volar radial cortex to the dorsal lip. There is volar (palmar) and proximal displacement of the distal fracture fragment, consistent with a Smith's fracture (Type II). There is impaction of fracture fragments, resulting in mild radial shortening. In addition, there is a minimally displaced fracture through the base of the ulnar styloid process.

9. The normal parameters for the distal radius are as follows:
    i)   radial length: ~ 11mm higher than the base of the distal ulna;
    ii) radial inclination: ~22°;
    iii) palmar tilt: ~11°.
    This is commonly remembered as '11-22-11.' These parameters aid in determining the amount of deformation of a distal radius when fractured, and serve as baseline measurements for guiding reductions - both closed and open.

Management

All displaced distal radius fractures, regardless of the amount of comminution, should have a closed reduction in the ER. Bringing the joint closer to anatomic alignment helps decrease pain, can take pressure off the median nerve, can decrease swelling, and allow for easier operative fixation. Provided that adequate reduction is achieved, the patient can be placed in a Charnley splint and closely monitored for any displacement. Once swelling has decreased, the Charnley splint is converted to a short arm cast. The method of closed reduction is described below.

Dorsal angulation (traction method)

A hematoma block (or alternative appropriate block) is given to the patient. The patient is placed in finger traps for approximately 10-20 minutes to provide adequate axial traction. If no finger traps are available, axial traction can be applied by flexing the arm to 90°, tying a sheet over the distal humerus and pulling downward with the foot, while pulling upward on the wrist. To adequately radially deviate the wrist, traction should be held by pulling on the patient's thumb and index fingers. The step-off of the fracture should be felt for at the dorsum of the wrist for dorsally angulated fractures. The fracture should then be milked upwards and volarly. A Charnley splint is placed while the patient remains in finger traps or while traction is applied.

Dorsal angulation (manipulation method)

After providing appropriate pain relief the wrist is manipulated firstly by re-creating and over-

exaggerating the fracture deformity to release the dorsal soft tissue hinge before correcting the position by traction and reduction. It is very important to first hyper-increase the deformity, otherwise an adequate reduction will not be achieved.

Volar angulation

For volar angulation, the reduction maneuver is the same as that described above, except that the fracture is milked upwards and dorsally. These fractures are often more difficult to reduce than dorsally displaced fractures; they will be more stable and should be splinted in supination.

Stable fractures, once reduced, can be closely monitored. Unstable fractures will need operative fixation. Indications of instability/fractures more likely to require operative fixation are: a comminuted fracture, intra-articular extension, age >40, dorsal displacement, loss of radial height and inclination.

Options for operative fixation include:

◆   Locked volar plating. This has become the gold standard for operative care of distal radial fractures suitable for even dorsally displaced distal radius fractures. The Henry approach to the distal radius is used for exposure of the fracture.
◆   Percutaneous pinning. This method can be used in extra-articular fractures, and is commonly used in the pediatric population. The fracture is held in place by a Kirschner wire that is usually driven through the radial styloid and a dorsal intra-osseous wire (Kapangi technique).
◆   External fixation. This may be used for injuries that are unstable with a significant amount of swelling preventing immediate fixation, or for initial damage control of open fractures. Locked plating has now made this a rare procedure.

Fractures that are adequately reduced operatively are placed in a volar splint for comfort, and patients can begin range of motion as tolerated on the first postoperative day. Those injuries that are casted are usually kept immobile in a cast for approximately six weeks before adequate healing is observed.

Key points

♦ When evaluating fractures of the distal radius, remember the rule: '11-22-11': radial height, inclination, palmar tilt.

♦ It is important to identify the following radiographically: angulation, comminution, intra-articular extension, any associated fractures, loss of radial height, inclination, or tilt.

♦ Closed reduction should be attempted on most displaced fractures.

♦ Pain that is difficult to control may be a sign of acute carpal tunnel syndrome, and may necessitate intervention sooner rather than later.

References

1. Putman MD, Seitz WH. Fractures of the distal radius. In: *Rockwood and Green's Fractures of Adults*. Bucholz RW, Heckman JD, Eds. Philadelphia, PA: Lippincott Williams & Wilkins, 2001: 815-67.

2. Fractures of the distal radius. In: *Operative Orthopaedics*, 2nd ed. Chapman MW, Ed. Philadelphia, PA: JB Lippincott, 1993: 1351-61.

3. Wood MB, Berquist TH. The hand and wrist. In: *Imaging of Orthopedic Trauma*. Berquist TH. New York, NY: Raven Press, 1992: 749-870.

Case 5

Clinical presentation

A 32-year-old woman is learning how to skateboard. She falls onto her right elbow during a jump off some steps. She presents to the ER for further evaluation.

Physical examination

There is gross deformity and swelling of the right elbow with pain on any attempted movement including supination and pronation. Distally, she has palpable radial and ulnar pulses. She can abduct her fingers, make an OK sign, and retropulse her thumb. Sensation is intact on the dorsum of her hand, tips of her fingers, and over the lateral side of her small finger.

Review the images below [Figures 14 and 15]. Describe your findings.

Questions

1. What is the diagnosis?

2. What is the mechanism of injury?

3. How are these injuries classified?

4. What is significant about the radial head in this particular injury pattern?

5. Which injury typically has nerve involvement, and which nerve is involved?

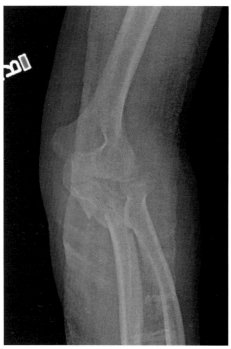

Figure 14.

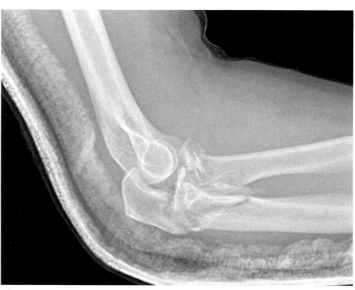

Figure 15.

Radiology findings

There are comminuted fractures of the proximal ulna and coronoid process, with an associated radial head fracture with subsequent lateral subluxation. There is intra-articular extension of the radial head and proximal ulna fractures.

Answers

1. Type III Monteggia variant fracture of the right elbow.

2. These injuries are caused by various means, each mechanism producing a different fracture pattern. The classification system is based on these patterns. The above fracture pattern has lateral subluxation of the radial head, with a fracture into the proximal ulnar shaft. This fracture is likely due to forced abduction of the elbow, levering the radial head out laterally as it contacts the proximal ulna, and fracturing the proximal ulna as the force is transmitted from the proximal radius to the ulna.

3. Monteggia fractures are classified using the Bado classification system. This system describes the injury based on the mechanism that produces it. The description is based on the location of the radial head with respect to the proximal ulna. The Bado classification consists of four types of fractures; however, in reality, there are multiple variants to this framework, as in the case above:
   i) Type I: radial head is dislocated anteriorly and the proximal ulna shaft fracture is angulated anteriorly. This is seen in a fracture caused by forced forearm pronation;
   ii) Type II: the radial head is dislocated posteriorly and the proximal ulna shaft fracture is angulated posteriorly. This is caused by an axial load applied to a forearm with a flexed elbow;
   iii) Type III: the radial head is dislocated laterally or anterolaterally with a non-angulated fracture of the proximal ulna. This is caused by forced abduction of the elbow, as in the case above;

   iv) Type IV: the radial head is dislocated anteriorly, combined with an anteriorly angled fracture of the ulnar shaft and radial shaft. This is caused by the same mechanism as a Type I fracture - forced forearm pronation.

4. The ulna fracture should be addressed first, because attempting to relocate the radial head first would be unsuccessful. In Monteggia fractures, reduction of the ulna shaft usually leads to automatic reduction of the radial head and operative reduction and fixation is required. Therefore, the ulna should be reduced and fixed first, and the radial head should then reduce. If it does not, the most common reason is a failure to accurately reduce the ulna which may need revision.

5. Type II Bado fractures usually have an associated posterior interosseous nerve/radial nerve injury.

Management

These fractures are treated operatively. The ulna shaft is reduced and held, usually with a plate. The radius should spontaneously reduce. If not, the reduction of the ulna should be carefully examined and corrected if not anatomic. Persistent dislocation of the intact radial head is rare but occasionally the annular ligament may block reduction. If the radial head is fractured, it may need to be repaired or a prosthetic replacement may be nececssary to restore elbow stability.

Key points

- A Monteggia fracture is a fracture/dislocation of the radial head, with an associated proximal ulna fracture.
- Monteggia fractures are classified based on the Bado classification system.
- The radial head usually spontaneously reduces after fixation of the ulna.
- Type II Bado fractures are sometimes associated with radial nerve injuries.

References

1. Bado JL. The Monteggia lesion. *Clin Orthop Relat Res* 1967; 50: 71-86.

2. Penrose JH. The Monteggia fracture with posterior dislocation of the radial head. *J Bone Joint Surg* 1951; 33B: 65-73.

3. Anderson LE, Meyer FN. Fractures of the shafts of the radius and ulna. In: *Fractures in Adults*, vol 1, 3rd ed. Rockwood CA, Green DP, Bucholz R, Eds. Philadelphia, PA: JB Lippincott, 1991.

4. Jessing P. Monteggia lesions and their complicating nerve damage. *Acta Orthop Scand* 1975; 46(4): 601-9.

5. Speed JS, Boyd HB. Treatment of fractures of the ulna with dislocation of the head of the radius. *JAMA* 1940; 115: 1699-704.

6. Papavasiliou VA, Nenopoulos SP. Monteggia-type elbow fractures in childhood. *Clin Orthop* 1988; 233: 230-3.

Chapter 5

Hand

Case 1

Clinical presentation

A 26-year-old man presents to the ER 24 hours after he was thrown off his bicycle as he tried to avoid a car. He landed on his left arm and describes an isolated injury to the left wrist only. He initially went home, but now presents because the swelling and pain have worsened.

Physical examination

There is some local swelling on the radial side of the wrist, tenderness to palpation in the anatomic snuff box, and particular pain with axial loading of the wrist. There are no vascular or sensory deficits. Motor examination is difficult to determine due to the patient's pain.

Review the image below [Figure 1]. Describe your findings.

Questions

1. What is the diagnosis?

2. What is the mechanism of injury?

3. How are these injuries classified?

4. What are the potential complications of this injury?

5. What other associated injuries can occur?

6. If initial plain films are negative, what measures can be taken to better visualize the affected bone? What other imaging modalities can assist in diagnosis?

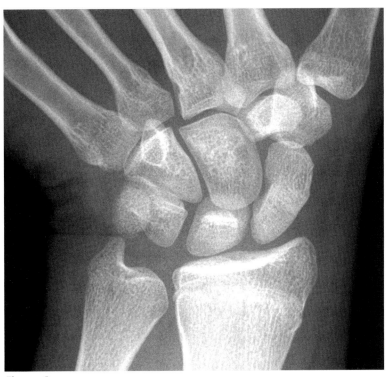

Figure 1.

Radiology findings

A plain film view of the left hand demonstrates an incomplete fracture line through the waist of the scaphoid without intra-articular extension. There is no displacement of fracture fragments. There is no evidence of a scapholunate dissociation or carpal instability.

Answers

1. Non-displaced fracture of the scaphoid waist (A2 according to the Herbert and Fisher system).

2. Scaphoid fractures most commonly occur in young adults after a fall onto the dorsiflexed, outstretched hand (also known as a FOOSH - Fall Onto OutStretched Hand).

3. Scaphoid fractures can be classified according to a number of systems. The most useful is the descriptive system, dividing fractures into those occurring in the distal pole or tuberosity, the proximal pole or the waist. Herbert and Fisher also classified scaphoid fractures into a system that predicts those fractures which require operative fixation [Figure 2, Table 1]. Stable, acute fractures are grouped as Type A injuries, whereas unstable, acute fractures are grouped as Type B injuries. This system also describes delayed union (Type C) and non-union (Type D) injuries.

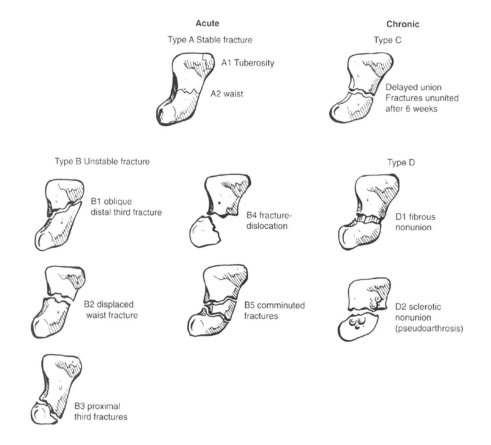

Figure 2. Herbert and Fisher's classification of fractures of the scaphoid. *Reprinted with permission from Lippincott Williams & Wilkins, © 2006. From Bucholz RW, Heckman JD, Court-Brown CM, et al, Eds. Rockwood and Green's Fractures in Adults, 6th ed. Philadelphia, PA: Lippincott Williams & Wilkins, 2006: 871.*

Table 1. Herbert and Fisher's classification of fractures of the scaphoid.

Type A	Acute (stable)	A1	Tubercle fracture
		A2	Non-displaced incomplete fracture of the waist
Type B	Acute (unstable)	B1	Oblique, distal third fracture
		B2	Displaced, complete fracture involving the waist
		B3	Fracture of the proximal pole
		B4	Fracture-dislocation pattern (trans-scaphoid perilunate dislocation)
		B5	Comminuted
Type C	Delayed union		
Type D	Non-union	D1	Fibrous non-union
		D2	Sclerotic non-union (pseudo-arthrosis)

4. Prompt diagnosis of scaphoid fractures is important. A delay in diagnosis can result in non-union, osteonecrosis, and post-traumatic arthritis. Osteonecrosis is a major concern due to the blood supply of the scaphoid [Figures 3 and 4]. The majority of the blood supply to the bone enters through the distal one third via scaphoid branches of the radial artery. A fracture can compromise vascular supply to the proximal pole, which is the most likely region of the scaphoid to be affected. Other

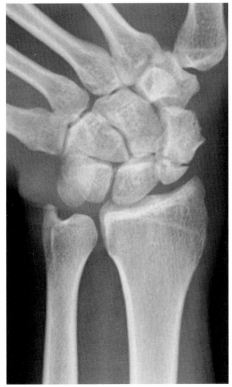

Figure 3. An obvious fracture of the proximal scaphoid is noted with patchy increased density of the proximal fragment. The smooth, sclerotic margins at the fracture line indicate non-union.

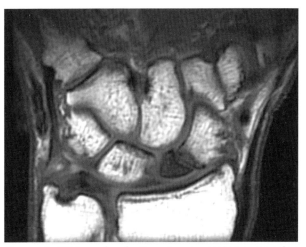

Figure 4. MR imaging further demonstrates avascular necrosis of the proximal scaphoid.

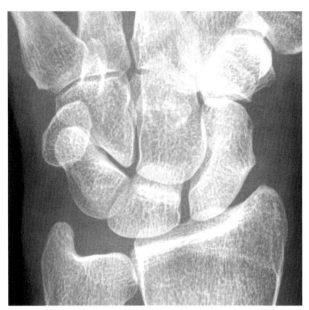

Figure 5. AP radiograph of the left wrist of a 26-year-old female after a fall onto an outstretched hand reveals no abnormalities.

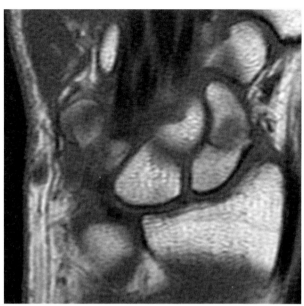

Figure 6. Coronal T1-weighted images of the same patient shows central marrow edema within the scaphoid, as well as an incomplete scaphoid waist fracture line.

complications include delayed union, wrist instability and reflex sympathetic dystrophy. Displaced scaphoid fractures may also be associated with a dorsal lunate tilt indicating dorsal intercalated segment instability (DISI).

5. Associated injuries often include a distal radius fracture, and/or a perilunate dislocation.

6. Scaphoid fractures may be very difficult to see on initial plain films [Figure 5]. Subtle signs such as a displaced fat pad may assist in diagnosis. In difficult cases, special scaphoid views of the wrist can be obtained, in which the scaphoid is visualized 'in profile' with the wrist in maximal ulnar deviation. Alternatively, in cases of high clinical suspicion, CT imaging or MRI may be of value in diagnosing occult fractures [Figure 6].

Management

The classification system for scaphoid fractures is helpful in the management:

◆ Type A fractures: placed in a short arm cast or scaphoid (thumb spica) cast for 8-12 weeks. Frequent follow-up with the orthopedic surgeon and repeat X-rays are required. A CT scan may also be required to evaluate any displacement in order to determine if definitive fixation is required.
◆ Type B fractures: initially splinted in a cast or thumb spica splint. Definitive fixation is required.
◆ Type C (delayed union), Type D (fibrous union): although rarely seen in the acute setting, they also require definitive fixation.

The usual method of definitive fixation is screw fixation.

Key points

♦ Scaphoid fractures may be easily missed on plain films and should be suspected if symptoms persist. In cases of high clinical suspicion, repeat imaging in ten days is needed. If an acute diagnosis is warranted, further evaluation with a CT or MRI should be considered.

♦ The majority of fractures occur in the middle third, or the waist, or the scaphoid.

♦ The blood supply of the scaphoid is key. The distal third has good blood supply from the dorsal scaphoid branch of the radial artery, and the proximal third is covered in cartilage and receives its blood supply through the bone. This blood supply will be disrupted by fracture.

♦ Examination of the surrounding carpal bones is important to avoid missing a perilunate dislocation. Missing this can be very easy, and should be suspected if the carpus just does not look right! The continuity of the carpal rows should be assessed. A comparative view of the other side may be useful.

References

1. Eisenhauer MA. Wrist & Forearm. In: *Emergency Medicine: Concepts and Clinical Practice*, 5th ed. Rosen P, *et al*, Eds. St. Louis, MO: Mosby-Year Book, 2002: 535-9.

2. Russe O. Fractures of the carpal navicular. *J Bone Joint Surg [Am]* 1960; 42: 759-68.

3. Bucholz RW, Heckman JD, Court-Brown CM, *et al*, Eds. *Rockwood and Green's Fractures in Adults*, 6th ed. Philadelphia, PA: Lippincott Williams & Wilkins, 2006.

4. Herbert TJ, Fisher WE: Management of the fractured scaphoid using a new bone screw. *J Bone Joint Surg Br* 1984; 66(1): 114-23.

5. Russe O. Fracture of the carpal navicular. Diagnosis, non-operative treatment, and operative treatment. *Am J Orthop* 1960; 42-A: 759-68.

Case 2

Clinical presentation

A 42-year-old man is thrown off his motorcycle when he skids over an icy bridge. He is wearing his helmet and well padded gear. His trauma workup in the ER is essentially negative. He has road rash on both his lower extremities and minor scrapes and bruises. He also is complaining of pain in his left hand, and subsequent X-rays are obtained.

Physical examination

On exam, the skin is intact. The dorsum of the wrist is swollen and tender to palpation over the hypothenar and thenar eminences. There is also tenderness just over Lister's tubercle. The patient has pain with flexion and extension of the wrist, as well as radial and ulnar deviation of the wrist. He has weak grip strength secondary to pain. Sensation is intact in the radial, median, and ulnar nerve distributions. The patient is able to abduct his fingers, retropulse his thumb, and

make an OK sign, but he does so with difficulty secondary to pain.

Review the images below [Figures 7 and 8]. Describe your findings.

Questions

1. What is the diagnosis?

2. What is the mechanism of injury?

3. What are Gilula's lines?

4. How are these injuries classified?

5. What is the 'spilled tea cup' sign?

6. Why is the lunate called the carpal keystone?

7. What is a VISI? What is a DISI?

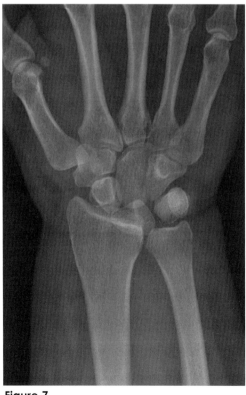

Figure 7.

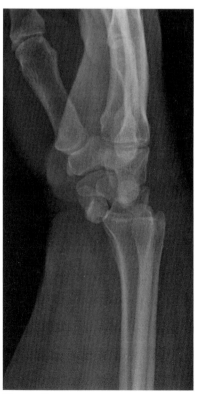

Figure 8.

Radiology findings

There is dislocation of the lunate from the proximal row of the carpal bones in a volar direction into the carpal canal. On the frontal radiograph, there is a triangular configuration of the lunate (normally appears quadrangular) and disruption of the proximal and middle carpal arcs (Gilula's lines). The triangular configuration is essentially pathognomonic for this injury. On the lateral radiograph, there is volar dislocation of the lunate relative to the articular surface of the distal radius, and the capitate has dropped to occupy the normal position of the lunate. The normal alignment between the distal radius, lunate, capitate and third metacarpal is lost [Figures 9 and 10]. The concave surface of the lunate has rotated by approximately 90° and now faces volarly (sometimes referred to as the 'spilled teacup sign'). The dislocated lunate lies volar to the carpal bones.

Answers

1. Lunate dislocation (stage IV carpal instability).

2. This injury usually occurs after forceful hyperextension of the wrist. An axial load is applied radially through the thenar eminence, forcing the wrist into extension. This usually causes damage to the radioscapholunate ligament (resulting in widening of the scapholunate interval on a radiograph). The scaphoid which bridges the proximal and distal carpal rows, has to be fractured or partly dislocated, causing instability between the two rows. With the force of this injury, the scaphoid

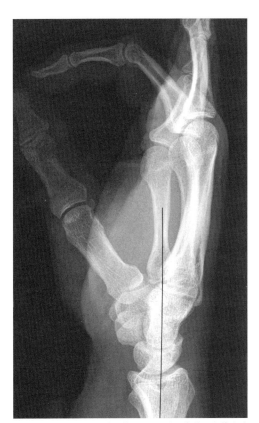

Figure 9. Normal alignment of the distal radius, lunate and capitate as seen on a lateral radiograph.

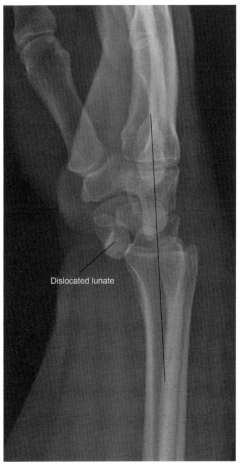

Dislocated lunate

Figure 10. Lunate dislocation is best identified on a lateral radiograph, where there is volar displacement of the lunate and disruption of the normal alignment between the distal radius, lunate and capitate.

can fracture with the proximal pole moving with the lunate. As the injury occurs, the force is transmitted through the space of Poirier - an area of weakness between the capitate and lunate because there are no supportive ligaments attaching here. The force continues to travel ulnarly until it disrupts the lunotriquetral articulation, injuring the radiolunotriquetral ligament. As the force travels ulnarly, the lunate will dislocate. This progression is known as Mayfield's progression of injury.

3. Gilula's lines are three smooth lines that can be drawn on an AP view of the normal wrist. A disruption of these lines indicates ligamentous instability, which is often better appreciated on a lateral radiograph. These lines are drawn along the proximal and distal surfaces of the proximal carpal row and the proximal cortical margins of the capitate and hamate [Figure 11].

4. A lunate dislocation is classified based on associated joints involved/ligaments injured. This correlates with the stage of Mayfield's progression of injury. The higher the classification, it is likely that a greater number of carpal ligaments/joints are injured and, therefore, there is greater progression of force through the wrist. Stage I disease involves the scapholunate joint. The injured ligaments are the radioscapholunate and interosseous scapholunate ligament. This can cause a widening of the scapholunate interval or a fracture through the scaphoid. As the scaphoid is injured, the carpal rows are affected. In Stage II, the radioscaphocapitate ligament is injured, which indicates injury to the capitolunate joint, a midcarpal joint. In Stage III, the distal radiolunotriquetral ligament is injured, which occurs as the force travels ulnarly. Finally, in Stage IV, the radiolunate joint is disrupted as the dorsal radiolunotriquetral ligament is disrupted, causing volar dislocation of the lunate. When a lunate dislocation is associated with a scaphoid fracture, this is known as a trans-scaphoid perilunate dislocation [Figures 12 and 13].

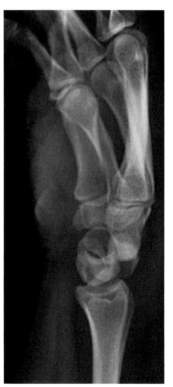

Figure 12. A lateral view of the hand demonstrates a displaced fracture of the scaphoid waist with dorsal displacement of the distal carpal row, as well as dorsal displacement of the capitate relative to the lunate. The lunate remains in articulation with the distal radius.

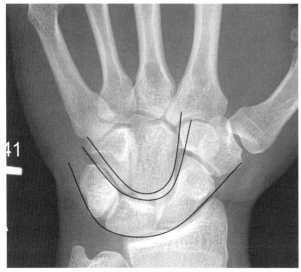

Figure 11. Normal AP radiograph of the hand demonstrating Gilula's arcs (lines).

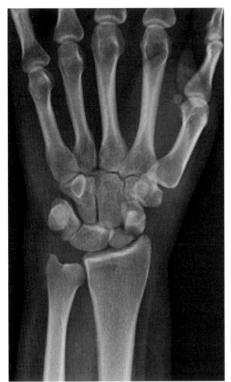

Figure 13. Frontal radiograph after reduction clearly demonstrates the associated scaphoid fracture.

5. On a lateral view, with a volar lunate dislocation, the volar tilt of the lunate often looks like a spilled teacup. Hence, a positive 'spilled tea cup' sign indicates a volar lunate dislocation.

6. The lunate is called the carpal keystone because it is a key to carpal stability. It is connected to both the scaphoid and the triquetrum. The scaphoid, due to its 45° obliquity, tends to flex when an axial compression force is applied; this force is transmitted through the lunate by the scapholunate ligament, in turn causing the lunate to flex. The triquetrum extends when axial load is applied to it, and this force is transmitted to the lunate by the lunotriquetral ligament, causing the lunate to extend. The lunate is thus the balance between flexion and extension of the proximal carpal row. Damage to the attaching ligaments causes an imbalance between flexion and extension of the carpus, and hence carpal instability.

7. VISI: with damage to the lunotriquetral ligament, the lunate will flex due to the unopposed pull of the scapholunate ligament. With a position of flexion >15°, the lunate becomes statically fixed, and volar intercalated static instability (VISI) results.

   DISI: with damage to the scapholunate ligament, there is unopposed extension on the lunate. When it flexes to >10°, it can also become statically fixed, and dorsal intercalated segment instability (DISI) results.

   These deformities affect radial and ulnar deviation of the wrist, as well as place mechanical disadvantages to flexion and extension.

Management

Closed reduction is initially attempted in the ER. Longitudinal traction is applied to the wrist. For the volar lunate dislocation above, the lunate is pushed dorsally, and counter pressure is applied volarly on the wrist. The wrist is then flexed and extended to reduce the capitate and lunate. If closed reduction fails, an urgent open reduction and stabilization is required.

Once swelling decreases, surgical correction is undertaken. These dislocations are considered emergencies due to the potential for carpal instability if not adequately corrected. If there are signs of a median nerve neuropathy, the patient's wrist should be reduced, stabilized and the carpal canal decompressed urgently.

In terms of operative fixation, if there is a good closed reduction of the lunate, the carpus is percutaneously pinned to the radius. The triquetrum and scaphoid are also percutaneously pinned to the lunate. If closed reduction is not successful, an open reduction is performed. If there is an associated scaphoid fracture, this is also fixed, usually with a dorsal approach and cannulated screw fixation.

Key points

- The lunate is known as the carpal keystone due to its function in proximal row stability.
- Perilunate fractures/dislocations follow a specific progression of injury, known as the Mayfield progression. The specific ligaments and joints injured correlate with the progression of the injury.
- If possible urgent closed reduction should be attempted, with conscious sedation, in the ER.
- These reductions are monitored closely for any residual deformity, and if closed reduction in the ER is unsuccessful, the patient should be taken to the operating theater.

References

1. Mayfield JK, Kilcoyne RK, Johnson RP. Carpal dislocations: pathomechanics and progressive perilunate instability. *J Hand Surg* 1980; 5: 226-41.

2. Johnson RP. The acutely injured wrist and its residuals. *Clin Orthop* 1980; 149: 33-44

3. Meyer S. Radiographic evaluation of wrist trauma *Semin Roentgen* 1991; 26(4): 300-17.

4. Bucholz RW, Heckman JD, Court-Brown CM, *et al*, Eds. *Rockwood and Green's Fractures in Adults*, 6th ed. Philadelphia, PA: Lippincott Williams & Wilkins, 2006.

5. Koval KJ, Zuckerman JD. *Handbook of Fractures*, 3rd ed. Philadelphia, PA: Lippincott Williams & Wilkins, 2006.

Case 3

Clinical presentation

A 36-year-old man was walking in the icy weather and slipped on the ice landing on his right hand. He presents to the ER complaining of pain at the base of his right palm.

Physical examination

There is swelling on the volar aspect of the patient's hand over the hypothenar area. The skin is intact. The patient has tenderness most pronounced over the ulnar aspect of his wrist. He has pain particularly when the wrist is extended. This is relieved somewhat with wrist hyperflexion. There are no neurovascular deficits.

Review the images below [Figures 14 and 15]. Describe your findings.

Questions

1. What is the diagnosis?

2. What is the mechanism of injury?

3. List some complications of this injury if left untreated.

4. What two important structures run medial to the pisiform? What important ligaments attach to the pisiform?

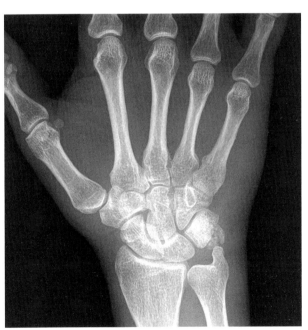

Figure 14.

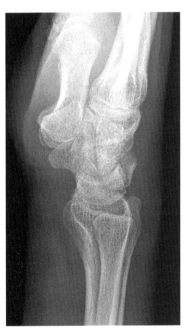

Figure 15.

Radiology findings

There is a minimally displaced fracture of the pisiform. The remaining carpal bones are unremarkable.

Answers

1. Pisiform fracture.

2. Fractures of the pisiform may occur secondary to direct trauma to the ulnar aspect of the wrist. They are also seen after forced hyperextension of the wrist joint, such as a fall onto the outstretched hand.

3. Failure to treat a pisiform fracture can result in delayed union, malunion or non-union. Patients may suffer from chronic pain, osteoarthritis, limitation of movement, a weak grip, subluxation, and later, pisotriquetral chondromalacia. Hence, if there is clinical suspicion for a fracture of the pisiform and plain films are negative, an MRI should be obtained for evaluation.

4. The ulnar nerve and artery run medial to the pisiform within Guyon's canal. A significantly displaced fracture can rarely result in injury to these structures. Ligament attachments to the pisiform include the flexor carpi ulnaris tendon, the flexor and extensor retinaculum, the pisometacarpal ligament, the pisohamate ligament and the abductor digiti quinti muscle. The patient will experience pain with extension of the wrist as the flexor carpi ulnaris is stressed over the fracture; this pain will be relieved with flexion as stress is taken off the tendon over the bone.

Management

Minimally displaced fractures, such as in the patient in this case, can be treated with immobilization using a short arm cast for 4-6 weeks. For displaced fractures, these can also be immobilized and allowed to heal. Operative fixation is not practical in this very small bone. If non-union occurs the loose fragment is excised. In the acute setting if the fragment is particularly painful it can also be excised without a trial of six weeks of immobilization.

Key points

- Isolated pisiform fractures are rare and usually occur in conjunction with fractures of other carpal bones or the distal radius.
- MRI is a valuable imaging modality in cases of a high index of suspicion but with negative plain films.
- In 50% of cases, a fractured pisiform is associated with fractures of other carpal bones or the distal radius.
- These fractures can be treated with immobilization. If non-union occurs, or the patient is particularly in pain, the fracture fragment can be excised.

References

1. Altinok MT, Ertem K, Sigirci A, Alkan A. An isolated acute pisiform fracture: usefulness of MR imaging. *The Internet Journal of Radiology* 2004; 3(2).

Case 4

Clinical presentation

A 36-year-old man was walking and slipped on the ice, landing on his left hand. He presents to the ER with pain on the back of his hand.

Physical examination

There is some swelling on the back of the left hand. The skin is intact, and there is no gross deformity of the wrist. The patient is mostly tender on the dorso-ulnar aspect of the hand, and has marked pain with wrist range of motion, most noted when his left wrist is ulnarly deviated. There are no neurovascular deficits.

Review the images below [Figures 16 and 17]. Describe your findings.

Questions

1. What is the diagnosis?

2. What is the mechanism of injury?

3. Which ligament is most commonly involved?

4. If there is high clinical suspicion, and the available AP and lateral views of the wrist are not helpful, what additional view can be obtained to better visualize the involved bone?

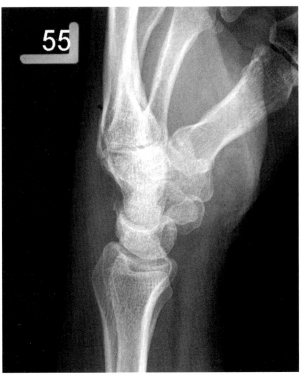

Figure 16.

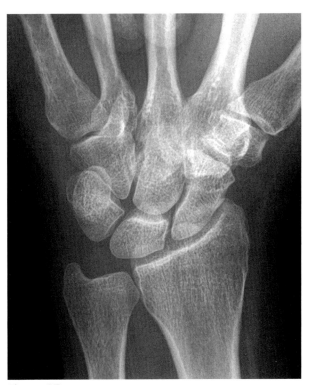

Figure 17.

Radiology findings

A lateral image of the left hand shows a small bone fragment located dorsally, consistent with an avulsion fracture of the triquetrum.

Answers

1. Fracture of the triquetrum.

2. These fractures are mostly avulsion injuries caused as the affected hand is hyper-extended and ulnarly deviated, the ulnar styloid hits the triquetrum, and a piece of the dorsum of the triquetrum is avulsed off. It is essentially a dorsal wrist sprain with avulsion of a small piece of bone with the capsular injury.

3. The fracture line most commonly involves the radiocarpal ligament.

4. The lunate is superimposed on the triquetrum, and can make a dorsally displaced fragment difficult to see on a lateral view. This same fragment can also be difficult to see on the AP view due to the overlying intact triquetrum. To isolate the dorsum of the triquetrum, an oblique view, with the wrist pronated can be diagnostic for an avulsion fracture.

Management

Dorsal avulsion fractures, or minimally displaced fractures, can be treated with simple splintage while painful.

Key points

♦ Lateral radiographs are often diagnostic of triquetral avulsion fractures, showing a bone fragment displaced dorsally.

♦ Triquetral fractures are rarely associated with perilunate dislocations.

♦ Management of these fractures involves immobilization while symptomatic.

References

1. Smith DK, Murray PM. Avulsion fractures of the volar aspect of triquetral bone of the wrist: a subtle sign of carpal ligament injury. *AJR Am J Roentgenol* 1996; 166(3): 609-14.

2. Letts M, Esser D. Fractures of the triquetrum in children. *J Pediatr Orthop* 1993; 13(2): 228-31.

Case 5

Clinical presentation

A 29-year-old man involved in a fist fight presents to the ER with pain and swelling at the base of his thumb.

Physical examination

On exam, there is swelling and pain at the base of his thumb. He resists local movement and the base of the thumb feels unstable. There is no abnormality of circulation or sensation and no pain with range of motion of his wrist. There is no pain, swelling, or deformity in his other digits.

Review the image below [Figure 18]. Describe your findings.

Questions

1. What is the diagnosis?

2. What is the mechanism of injury?

3. What muscles cause displacement of the fragments?

4. What are some prognostic factors for these injuries?

5. What types of complications may occur?

6. What is a similar comminuted fracture across the base of the first metacarpal called?

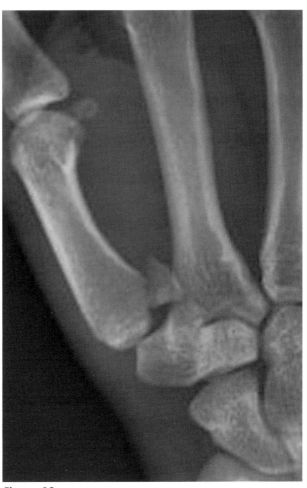

Figure 18.

Radiology findings

There is an oblique intra-articular fracture of the volar-ulnar aspect of the first metacarpal base that extends into the first carpometacarpal joint. A small triangular fragment of the base of the first metacarpal remains in articulation with the trapezium. This fragment involves approximately 40% of the articular surface with a step-off of approximately 6mm.

Answers

1. Bennett fracture [Figure 19].

2. A Bennett fracture (better known as a fracture-dislocation) occurs due to forced abduction of the thumb, such as that seen in fist fights.

3. The adductor pollicis causes proximal migration of the proximal phalanx, and the abductor pollicis longus causes rotational deformity by flexion and supination (Table 2).

4. Poor prognostic indicators include fractures with shearing injury to the radial side of the articular surface of the trapezium, significant fracture displacement and impaction at the carpometacarpal joint.

5. A Bennett fracture is a serious injury, and delay in treatment can result in an increased incidence of potential complications. If not treated, chronic instability and pain will occur.

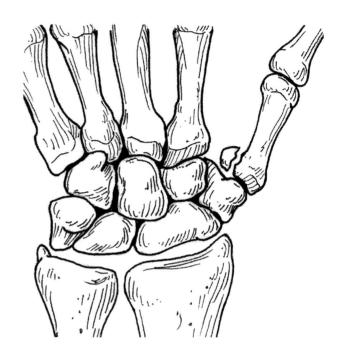

Figure 19. Depiction of a Bennett fracture - an intra-articular fracture-dislocation at the base of the thumb. *Reprinted with permission from the Radiological Society of North America. Hunter T, Peltier L, Lund P. Musculoskeletal eponyms: who are those guys? Radiographics 2000; 20(3): 819-36.*

Table 2. Muscle function.

Muscle	Origin	Attachment	Function	Innervation
Adductor pollicis	Two heads attach from the shaft of the third metacarpal and capitate	Base of the proximal phalanx of the thumb	Thumb adduction	Ulnar n.
Abductor pollicis longus	Posterior radius and ulna shaft	Base of the first metacarpal	Thumb extension and abduction	Radial nerve PIN

Other complications include damage to the local sensory branches of the radial nerve. Long-term complications include osteoarthritis, loss of thumb movements, and joint stiffness.

6. A comminuted fracture of the base of the first metacarpal is known as a Rolando fracture [Figure 20]. Its prognosis is worse than that of a Bennett fracture and it occurs after a greater force of injury.

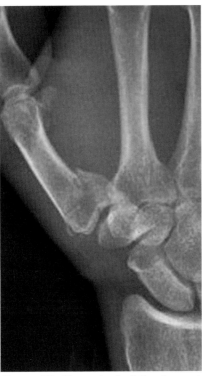

Figure 20. Comminuted fracture at the base of the first metacarpal, known as a Rolando fracture.

Management

Both Rolando and Bennet fractures are intra-articular fractures, and should be treated operatively in order to adequately stabilize the joint. Immediately in the ER, the patient can be placed in a volar resting splint for comfort and stability. Operatively, these fractures can be treated with a closed reduction and percutaneous pinning using fluoroscopy.

Key points

◆ A Bennett fracture is an intra-articular fracture of the base of the first metacarpal, involving the first carpometacarpal joint.

◆ A Rolando fracture is a more comminuted Bennett fracture, and is a higher energy injury.

◆ They are both treated with closed reduction with percutaneous pinning.

◆ Damage to the dorsal sensory radial nerve is possible.

References

1. Hunter T, Peltier L, Lund P. Musculoskeletal eponyms: who are those guys? *Radiographics* 2000; 20(3): 819-36.

2. Koval KJ, Zuckerman JD. *Handbook of Fractures*, 3rd ed. Philadelphia, PA: Lippincott Williams & Wilkins, 2006.

3. Bucholz RW, Heckman JD, Court-Brown CM, *et al. Rockwood and Green's Fractures in Adults*, 6th ed. Philadelphia, PA: Lippincott Williams & Wilkins, 2006.

Case 6

Clinical presentation

A 26-year-old man presents to the ER with pain and swelling at the base of his small left finger. This happened after he punched another man in a drunken brawl.

Physical examination

There is swelling at the base of the left small finger and the knuckle is less prominent than on the right hand. The skin is intact and there are no fight bites on the knuckle. There is less than a two second capillary refill, and sensation is intact in the ulnar nerve distribution. The patient cannot extend at the metacarpophalangeal (MCP) joint.

Review the image below [Figure 21]. Describe your findings.

Questions

1. What is the diagnosis?

2. What is the mechanism of injury?

3. Do these injuries typically involve the articular surface?

4. Up to what degree of angulation of this injury is acceptable?

5. What is a fight bite?

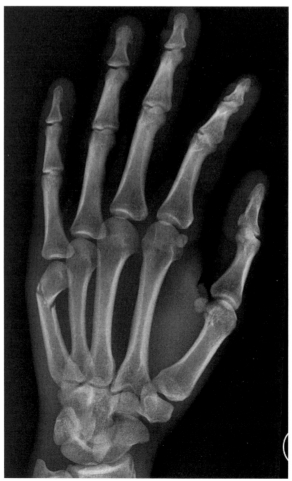

Figure 21.

Radiology findings

There is a transverse fracture of the neck of the fifth metacarpal with dorsal angulation of the distal fracture fragment. The angle of displacement of the distal fragment is 32° (the normal metacarpal neck angle is approximately 15°, and a measured angle of 47° is actually 32° of displacement). There is no intra-articular extension of the fracture line.

Answers

1. Fracture of the fifth metacarpal neck (Boxer's fracture).

2. Boxer's fractures occur commonly after direct trauma to the hand. The classic presentation is a patient presenting after punching something, or someone with a closed fist.

3. A classic Boxer's fracture does not involve the articular surface. However, an infrequent variant of a Boxer's fracture may occur, in which a fracture of the metacarpal head results in involvement of the joint space. These fractures may also be unstable and require operative fixation.

4. The acceptable degree of angulation of the distal fracture fragment varies according to the affected metacarpal. In the fifth metacarpal, volar angulation of up to 45° is acceptable. Slightly less angulation is tolerated in the fourth metacarpal, which is not as mobile as the fifth metacarpal. In the second and third metacarpals, angulation under 15° is tolerated; anything greater puts the patient at an increased risk of malunion. The more distally the fracture line occurs at the metacarpal neck, the greater the tolerated angulation.

5. A fight bite is a laceration over a joint in the hand. The laceration is curved, like the base of a tooth, and is assumed to be contaminated with oral flora. These patients need to be treated with broad spectrum antibiotics and the wound should be monitored closely.

Management

Most Boxer's fractures are treated with simple splintage until comfortable, followed by active mobilization. Commonly, the profile of the knuckle will be depressed but the hand will be fully functional. Reduction can be attempted, but holding the fracture in the reduced position is difficult and commonly the position is lost.

Closed reduction in the ER is done by applying pressure dorsally over the base of the fifth proximal phalanx/distal aspect of the fifth metacarpal. The patient can then be placed in an ulnar gutter splint in an intrinsic plus position. It is, however, difficult to apply a splint that will adequately hold the position, and if lost it may be decided to do a further closed reduction and add percutaneous pinning in the operating theater. For Boxer's fractures that involve the joint and are displaced or unstable, closed reduction should be attempted in the ER in order to align the fracture fragments as best as possible, and the patient should be scheduled for a closed reduction with percutaneous pinning.

Key points

♦ A Boxer's fracture is a transverse fracture of the metacarpal neck with volar angulation of the distal fracture fragment and is most commonly seen in the fifth metacarpal.

♦ Most are treated non-operatively with a slight residual deformity but normal function.

♦ For Boxer's fractures that involve the joint, if a reduction is difficult to maintain, a closed reduction with percutaneous pinning may be indicated.

♦ The degree of acceptable angulation varies per digit, with the small finger able to accept the greatest amount of angulation.

References

1. Koval KJ, Zuckerman JD. *Handbook of Fractures*, 3rd ed. Philadelphia, PA: Lippincott Williams & Wilkins, 2006.
2. Bucholz RW, Heckman JD, Court-Brown CM, *et al. Rockwood and Green's Fractures in Adults*, 6th ed. Philadelphia, PA: Lippincott Williams & Wilkins, 2006.

Case 7

Clinical presentation

A 20-year-old, right-hand-dominant woman presents after her right hand became caught in her car door as it was closing. She notices immediate pain in her hand, between her thumb and index finger, and presents to the ER for further evaluation.

Physical examination

On physical exam there is swelling over the dorsum of the right hand, mostly on the radial aspect. There are some abrasions and lacerations, but they appear superficial and do not go down to bone. She has good sensation at the back of her hand and at the tips of her fingers, but is tender on the back of her hand. She has brisk capillary refill at the tip of the index finger. There is scissoring of the index finger over the long finger and attempted motion of the fingers is painful.

Review the images below [Figures 22 and 23]. Describe your findings.

Questions

1. What is the diagnosis?

2. With these injuries, what is the maximum angulation and shortening of the involved bone that is considered acceptable?

3. Describe the anatomy of the metacarpals.

4. List the potential complications of these injuries.

5. How does treatment for a short oblique fracture differ from a long oblique fracture in the metacarpals?

6. How are these injuries classified?

7. On physical examination, how would you assess for rotational abnormalities in this type of injury?

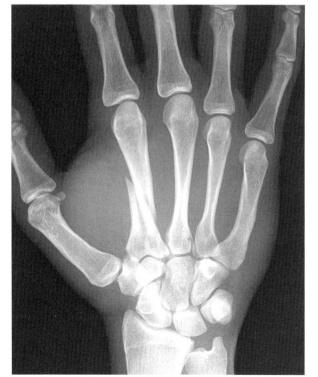

Figure 22.

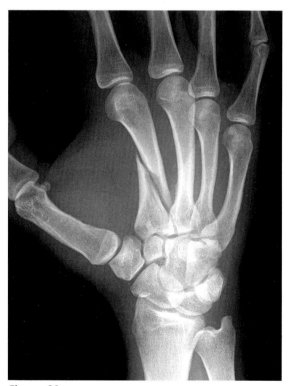

Figure 23.

Radiology findings

There is an oblique fracture involving the midshaft of the second metacarpal. It is classified as a long fracture, as the length of the fracture line is greater than twice the radial-ulnar diameter of the metacarpal. There is proximal and ulnar displacement of the distal fracture fragment. In addition, there is dorsal apex angulation noted of approximately 9° (occurring due to unbalanced intrinsic muscle forces). The head of the second metacarpal points volarly.

Answers

1. Long oblique fracture of the second metacarpal.

2. Metacarpal shaft fractures involving the second and third metacarpals typically allow for less than 10-15° of dorsal angulation and approximately 5mm shortening. Anything greater than these parameters increases the need for surgical management. These values differ for fractures in the fourth metacarpal, where up to 30-35° of angulation is accepted. In the small finger, up to 50° of angulation can be accepted. The normal neck to shaft angle in the metacarpals is 15° and must always be taken into account when determining the apex dorsal angulation. Despite these measured parameters, the critical operative indication is the presence of a rotational deformity that will make the fingers cross on attempted flexion and create a significant disability.

3. The index and middle fingers articulate with the capitate and trapezoid; these articulations have limited motion, which is why less deformity is acceptable with these two fingers. The small and ring fingers articulate with the hamate, and have more motion in their articulation with this bone. For this reason, a greater degree of deformity is allowed when these fingers are injured. There are three palmar and four dorsal interossei. They arise from the metacarpal shafts and insert into the extensor hood of the metacarpals. The palmar interossei adduct the fingers, the dorsal interossei abduct the fingers. The lumbricals attach from the flexor digitorum profundus on the radial side, and insert into the extensor hood. They flex the MCP joint and extend the interphalangeal joints. The interossei are supplied by the ulnar nerve. The radial two lumbricals are supplied by the median nerve, and the two ulnar lumbricals are supplied by the ulnar nerve. It is these muscles and tendons that create the dorsal angulation and rotation of a metacarpal shaft fracture.

4. Complications of a metacarpal shaft fracture include malunion, non-union, intrinsic/extrinsic tendon tightness, deformity, and persistent dorsal apex angulation.

5. Short oblique fractures often have less displacement than long oblique fractures and, therefore, are more amenable to closed treatment with reduction and splinting. Like long oblique fractures, however, they should be closely monitored clinically for rotational deformity and with weekly radiographs. If there is angulation or deformity beyond acceptable limits, then operative fixation may be indicated. The principles of fixation for short oblique fractures are the same as that for long oblique fractures.

6. Metacarpal shaft fractures can be classified according to the orientation of the fracture line: transverse, oblique, and spiral. Typically, direct or axial injuries result in transverse or oblique fractures, whereas torsion injuries result in spiral fractures.

7. It is most important to assess for a rotational deformity of a metacarpal shaft fracture; failure to recognize and fix this deformity will affect function. This assessment is best done clinically. Compare the injured and uninjured digits through a full range of motion by asking the patient to flex their fingers, or make a fist. Flexion should result in each digit pointing to the scaphoid tuberosity, and extension should result in each digit being parallel to the next as well as all the fingernails pointing in the same direction. If there is scissoring, or overlap of the digits, then there is rotational deformity. If the patient feels too much pain when actively making a fist,

then passive flexion and extension of the wrist will create some finger motion and may allow the examiner to pick up on any scissoring.

Management

The fracture should be closed reduced in the ER. For a metacarpal fracture, the hand can be splinted in the intrinsic plus position. This involves flexing the affected MCP joint ~70°, and keeping the interphalangeal joints in extension; this tightens the collateral ligaments and prevents lateral motion of the fracture fragment. It is very difficult for splintage to hold position if the fracture is unstable.

In this case, there is not much deformity of the affected fracture fragment, and no reduction is necessary. However, based on physical exam, this fracture is causing a rotational deformity, therefore, it requires surgical fixation. Options for surgical stabilization include the use of Kirschner wires (for an oblique fracture these should be placed perpendicular to the fracture line to prevent torsion or distraction deformity) or a formal ORIF with screws or plate fixation.

Key points

♦ Rotational deformity is the critical feature requiring reduction and operative intervention in metacarpal fractures.

♦ Varying degrees of angulation are acceptable for each digit. For the index and long fingers, 10-15° of angulation are acceptable, the ring finger, ~30° of angulation is acceptable, and in the small finger, up to 50° of angulation is acceptable. Rotation is not acceptable.

♦ Rotation can be assessed for by examining the fingers in both full extension and flexion.

♦ Metacarpal shaft fractures that are reduced should be splinted in the 'safe' position, or 'ulnar plus.' This involves flexion of the MCPs to 70-90°, and extension of the interphalangeal joints.

References

1.   Kozin SH, Thoder JJ, Lieberman G. Operative treatment of metacarpal and phalangeal shaft fractures. *J Am Acad Orthop Surg* 2000; 8: 111-21.

Case 8

Clinical presentation

A 26-year-old football player is hit on the left hand with the ball. He notes immediate pain and swelling of the left long and ring fingers and the inability to use them. He presents to the ER for further evaluation.

Physical examination

On exam, there is swelling over the dorsum of the left long and ring fingers. The skin is intact. They appear shortened compared with the right hand. There is brisk capillary refill at the apex of the affected digits, and sensation is intact to light touch at the apex of the affected digits.

Review the images below [Figures 24 and 25]. Describe your findings.

Questions

1. What is the diagnosis?

2. What is the mechanism of injury?

3. What complications can occur with this injury?

4. How are these injuries classified?

5. What should be looked for on a post-reduction lateral radiograph?

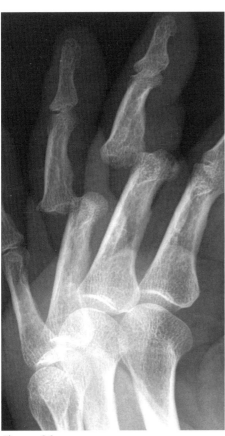

Figure 24.

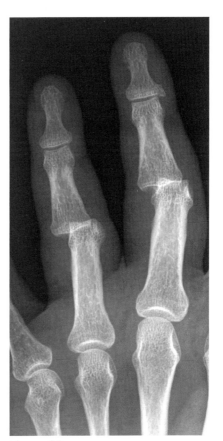

Figure 25.

Radiology findings

There is complete dorsal dislocation of the proximal interphalangeal (PIP) joints of both the long and ring digits. No fractures or loose bone fragments are identified.

Answers

1. Dorsal dislocation of the PIP joints of the long and ring digits.

2. Dislocation of the PIP joint occurs due to a hyperextension injury of the joint.

3. After management of this injury, patients may develop joint stiffness or post-traumatic osteoarthritis. In fracture-dislocations, residual joint instability may occur.

4. PIP joint dislocations can be classified into dorsal, pure volar and rotatory volar dislocations. They can also be classified into three groups:
    i)   Type I injuries are stable hyperextension injuries resulting in avulsion of the volar plate from the base of the middle phalanx. The joint surface is intact;
    ii) Type II injuries are stable dorsal dislocations with injury to a ligament;
    iii) Type III injuries are unstable dislocations with an associated fracture. The fracture may be stable (involving less than 40% of the base of the middle phalanx) or unstable (involving greater than 40% of the base). When the fracture fragment involves more than 40% of the base of the middle phalanx, there is a high incidence of injury to the lateral collateral ligament.

5. Persistent subluxation can be seen on post-reduction lateral radiographs in cases of dorsal dislocation. If there is residual subluxation, the affected digit should be splinted in extension rather than beginning range of motion.

Management

The affected joints need to be reduced. A local digital block is given, using lidocaine without epinephrine. For a dorsal dislocation, after the finger is anesthetized, force is applied in a volar direction to reduce the dislocated joint. Traction should NOT be applied when reducing. This is because the volar plate is involved in the injury. If traction is applied, this may allow for the volar plate to enter the joint space and cause continued subluxation of the distal interphalangeal joint (DIP), along with further damage to the volar plate. Once reduced, an immediate range of motion is begun, provided that no subluxation of the DIP is noted on post-reduction lateral radiographs. If there is subluxation, the affected joint is splinted in extension for 2-3 weeks.

Key points

- Dorsal dislocation of the proximal interphalangeal joint is more common than volar dislocation.
- Associated fractures of the base of the middle phalanx can result in an unstable injury.
- Congruence on the lateral X-ray is assessed to detect residual subluxation.
- To reduce a dorsal dislocation, volarly directed force is all that is required. Applying axial traction may involve the volar plate.

References

1. Otani K, Fukuda K, Hamanishi C. An unusual dorsal fracture-dislocation of the proximal interphalangeal joint. *J Hand Surg Eur Vol* 2007; 32(2): 193-4.

2. Wang QC, Johnson BA. Fingertip injuries. *Am Fam Physician* 2001; 63(10): 1961-6.

3. Freiberg A, Pollard BA, Macdonald MR, Duncan MJ. Management of proximal interphalangeal joint injuries. *Hand Clin* 2006; 22(3): 235-42.

Case 9

Clinical presentation

An 18-year-old male cricket player presents to the ER with right long finger pain and a deformity after catching a ball at a recent game.

Physical examination

There is gross deformity of the right long finger. There is some swelling over the distal phalanx. The skin is intact. The patient is unable to extend the DIP of the finger, and has pain with passive motion and when the examiner palpates over the DIP joint. Capillary refill and sensation are normal at the finger tip.

Review the images below [Figures 26 and 27]. Describe your findings.

Questions

1. What is the diagnosis?

2. What is the mechanism of injury?

3. What muscle group is involved in the abnormal deformity? Describe the anatomy of the extensor mechanism.

4. What secondary deformity may occur?

5. How are these injuries classified?

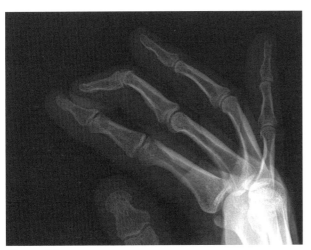

Figure 26.

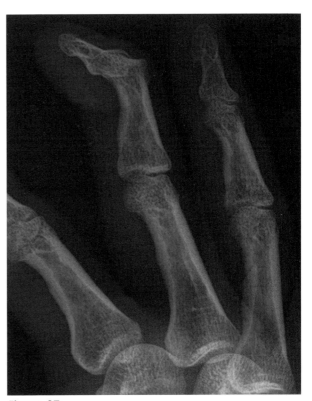

Figure 27.

Radiology findings

There is a flexion deformity of the DIP joint without evidence of a fracture. There is no volar subluxation of the DIP joint.

Answers

1. Tendinous mallet finger.

2. This injury results from hyperflexion to the DIP joint while it is in an extended position. It is commonly seen in athletes after attempting to catch a ball which hits the tip of the finger (baseball, cricket, volleyball). The sudden, forceful flexion of the distal fingertip causes a fracture, avulsion or tearing of the extensor tendon's insertion at the DIP. This allows for unopposed flexion, causing the deformity. A fragment of bone from the dorsum of the DIP may or may not be present. If an avulsion of bone is present, then the diagnosis is a bony mallet fracture.

3. Mallet deformities occur due to loss of the extensor mechanism of the DIP joint. There is a flexion deformity after the injury due to unopposed flexion by the flexor digitorum profundus. The extensor tendon courses over the dorsum of the digit. It trifurcates at the PIP joint, giving off a central tendon, and two branches off to either side of the digit. The central tendon called the central slip allows for extension of the PIP, as it attaches at the base of the PIP. The branches on either side of the digit are called the lateral bands. The lumbrical and interossei muscles also join the lateral bands, and this unit is called the conjoined lateral band as it continues distally. The conjoined lateral bands insert at the base of the distal phalanx and extend the DIP. With forced flexion, these conjoined lateral bands can be avulsed/torn/stretched, causing the mallet deformity.

4. A secondary 'swan neck' deformity can result. Here, flexion deformity of the DIP joint leads to unbalanced tone in the extensor mechanism and causes hyperextension at the PIP joint. With the lack of extension at the DIP, this results in a finger that looks like a swan's neck.

5. These injuries may involve the tendon (tendinous mallet finger) or bone (mallet fracture). Plain films are obtained to differentiate between the two types. An avulsion fracture may be seen at the base of the affected distal phalanx [Figure 28]. Mallet injuries can be classified according to Doyle's system (Table 3).

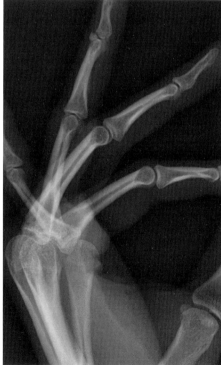

Figure 28. A lateral radiograph of the left hand demonstrates an avulsion fracture at the base of the distal phalanx of a digit in a 30-year-old male. This is consistent with a bony mallet finger without volar subluxation.

Table 3. Doyle's classification.

I	Closed tendon disruption
II	Open injury - laceration at DIP joint with tendon disruption
III	Open injury - deep abrasion with tissue and/or tendon loss

IV	Mallet fracture:
	    Type A: pediatric injury
	    Type B: 20-40% of articular surface involved in an adult
	    Type C: >50% of articular surface involved in an adult

Management

Mallet fingers can be classified as acute or chronic. Those that present within four weeks are acute injuries, and those that present after four weeks are chronic injuries. In this case, the patient has an acute injury. Management options are outlined below.

Acute

- Type I injuries: the DIP joint is splinted in extension. If a swan neck deformity is present, the DIP and PIP joint can be splinted. Splinting is done for approximiately 6-8 weeks, followed by splinting at night for two further weeks. For those patients that are unable to tolerate the splint for an extended period of time, a Kirschner wire can be used as an internal splint to hold the DIP in extension.
- Type II and III injuries: because these are open injuries, they require surgical repair of the tendon and thorough irrigation. Type III injuries may require multiple reconstructive procedures.
- Type IV injuries: these injuries can be treated conservatively or operatively. Extension splinting for 6-8 weeks can be done. Operative options include open versus closed reduction with percutaneous pinning.

Chronic

- Type I injuries: extension splinting for ten weeks, followed by two weeks of night-time splinting. If the patient is unhappy with the amount of extension that they have in their distal phalanx, surgery can be performed. Because these injuries are chronic, reconstruction of the tendon is often required. Various procedures can be performed to repair the extensor tendon, and then a percutaneous pin is placed to keep the DIP in extension for 6-8 weeks. If previous surgery has failed or the patient has pain in the affected digit due to a chronic mallet finger, then an arthrodesis of the DIP joint can be performed.
- Type II and III injuries: these are open injuries and, therefore, present in the acute setting rather than in the chronic setting.
- Type IV injuries: these are treated in a similar fashion to chronic Type I injuries, except, with the fracture fragment there may be non-union or malunion. For either of these injuries, re-reduction can be attempted, with fixation using a K-wire, screw, or tension band.

Key points

- A mallet finger is a hyperflexion deformity due to loss of the extensor mechanism of the DIP joint.
- Injuries may be tendinous or bony, and are classified according to the Doyle system.
- Volar subluxation of the distal phalanx is an important finding, as it may indicate the need for surgical management.
- These injuries can be treated non-surgically with splinting in extension for approximately eight weeks, if the patient is able to tolerate and be compliant with treatment.

References

1. Bendre AA, Hartigan BJ, Kalainov DM. Mallet finger. *Journal of the American Academy of Orthopedic Surgeons* 2005; 13: 336-44.
2. Doyle JR: Extensor tendons - acute injuries. In: *Operative Hand Surgery*, 3rd ed. Green DP, Ed. New York, NY: Churchill-Livingstone, 1993, 2: 1925-54.

Case 10

Clinical presentation

A 43-year-old, right-hand-dominant, male skier presents to the ER after falling onto an outstretched right hand while downhill skiing. He reports pain at the base of his right thumb that is preventing him from using it. Wrapping his hand around light objects such as a drinking glass or the steering wheel of his car causes him significant discomfort. He presents for further evaluation.

Physical examination

There is swelling noted at the ulnar aspect of the base of the right thumb. There is some ecchymosis, but the skin is intact. The patient has good sensation at the tip of his thumb and on the dorsum of his hand; he has normal circulation. The base of the thumb is not grossly deformed. His thumb is tender and he will not allow you to move his thumb. An intra-articular lidocaine injection is performed. The first digit MCP joint is stressed. You notice gross instability with valgus stress as the thumb appears to be abducted at the base greater than 30°. You compare this motion with the contralateral thumb,

and indeed note it to be increased on the injured side.

Review the images below [Figures 29 and 30]. Describe your findings.

Questions

1. What is the diagnosis?

2. What is the mechanism of injury?

3. What is a Stener lesion?

4. In the long term, what associated complications can occur?

5. What radiographic findings suggest a complete rupture of the involved ligament? What other findings might be seen on imaging?

6. Describe the anatomy of the MCP joint.

7. What nerve is at risk with operative fixation of this injury?

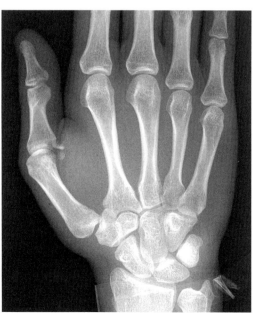

Figure 29.

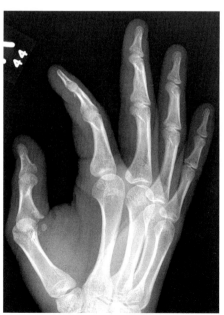

Figure 30.

Radiology findings

There is a small, non-displaced avulsion fracture at the ulnar aspect of the base of the proximal phalanx of the first digit. This is clearly identified on the oblique radiograph. There is no evidence of subluxation. This fracture is at the insertion site of the ulnar collateral ligament (UCL) on the MCP joint of the thumb, and is secondary to disruption of this ligament at this location. These findings are consistent with an avulsion fracture of the insertion of the UCL.

Answers

1. Gamekeeper's thumb (also called skier's thumb).

2. These injuries result from any type of valgus stress to the thumb. Commonly, they are due to a fall onto the outstretched hand with the thumb abducted in skiers (i.e. thumb caught in the pole strap of a ski pole). The valgus force is applied to an abducted thumb, and causes injury to the already stressed UCL.

3. A Stener lesion occurs when the UCL is ruptured. The torn end retracts and lies superficially to the adductor aponeurosis, which will prevent it from healing in the correct position. On physical examination, this may be palpated as a lump over the medial aspect of the MCP joint of the thumb.

4. There is an increased incidence of MCP joint arthritis. Patients with complete rupture of the UCL and with delayed repair have an increased incidence of instability, weakness, and pain on pinch grasp.

5. Findings to suggest a complete rupture include a minimum of 3mm volar subluxation of the phalanx on the metacarpal and a radial deviation of greater than 40° in extension and 20° in flexion. Radiographs may also depict findings compatible with rheumatoid arthritis, as these patients have a higher incidence of a gamekeeper's thumb than the general population.

6. The joint consists of a dorsal capsule and a volar plate, which attaches the metacarpal to the proximal phalanx. The radial and ulnar collateral ligaments arise from the metacarpal head, and attach to the lateral and medial aspect of the base of the proximal phalanx, respectively. The UCL is a strong structure, 6mm x 12mm in dimension, and when it is excessively strained it can cause an avulsion fracture at the base of the proximal phalanx, called a gamekeeper's fracture.

7. The sensory branch of the radial nerve is at risk with operative fixation.

Management

For such injuries where there is minimal instability of the affected MCP joint on physical exam, conservative management with a splint preventing abduction or adduction of the affected thumb is the means of treatment. The majority of such injuries, however, are treated operatively. An incision is made on the dorsal ulnar aspect of the thumb. The adductor aponeurosis is first encountered, followed by the dorsal capsule. The affected UCL is found displaced to the wrong side of the aponeurosis. It should then be reduced and repaired. In a chronic tear, the two ends of the capsule may not be found. In such a case, the end that is visible can be attached to the periosteum, or a tendon reconstruction using the palmaris longus can be performed. If there is a gamekeeper's fracture present, a small fragment may be removed, but a large fragment can be reduced and held in place with a Kirschner wire. The digit is then immobilized in a thumb spica splint or cast for approximiately four weeks, followed by range of motion training.

Key points

- A gamekeeper's thumb is due to partial or complete disruption of the UCL at the MCP joint of the thumb and may be associated with an avulsion fracture.

- Stener lesions will prevent appropriate healing of an UCL rupture and require operative repair. They may be palpable over the MCP joint of the thumb and occur due to rupture and displacement of the UCL.

- Most of these injuries are treated operatively. On initial presentation in the ER, the patient can be placed in a thumb spica splint and referred to a hand surgeon for early further care.

- To make the diagnosis, a stress test of the UCL is performed. If the patient is too tender to allow testing, consider using intra-articular lidocaine before stress testing.

References

1. Leggit JC, Meko CJ. Acute finger injuries: part II. Fractures, dislocations, and thumb injuries. *Am Fam Physician* 2006; 73(5): 827-34.

2. Campbell CS. Gamekeeper's thumb. *J Bone Joint Surg [Br]* 1955; 37-B(1): 148-9.

3. Stener B. Displacement of the ruptured ulnar collateral ligament of the metacarpo-phalangeal joint of the thumb. *J Bone Joint Surg [Br]* 1962; 44: 869-79.

Case 11

Clinical presentation

A 20-year-old soccer player is hit on his left small finger by the soccer ball during practice. He notes immediate pain at the tip of the finger, and is brought into the ER for further evaluation.

Physical examination

There is swelling and ecchymosis of the distal phalanx of the left small finger. The skin is intact, and there is no evidence of a nail bed injury or underlying hematoma. The patient has pain with palmar flexion of the DIP joint, and decreased sensation at the tip of the finger, likely due to the swelling and pain from the injury. There is brisk capillary refill.

Review the images below [Figures 31 and 32]. Describe your findings.

Questions

1. What is the diagnosis?

2. How do these injuries occur?

3. What is a common complication of this injury and how is it treated?

4. Why are these injuries usually stable?

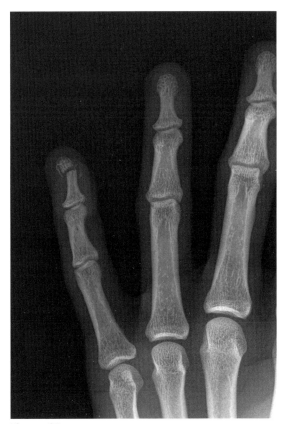

Figure 31.

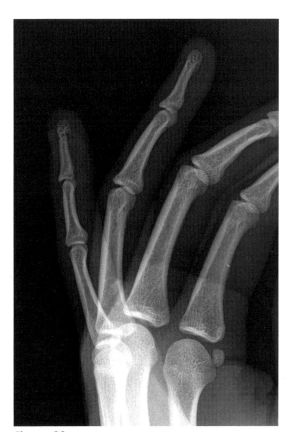

Figure 32.

Radiology findings

There is a transverse, comminuted fracture through the distal fifth phalangeal tuft. There is mild ulnar displacement of the distal fracture fragment. There is no irregularity of the adjacent soft tissues to suggest a skin laceration.

Answers

1. Tuft fracture of the fifth distal phalanx.

2. These fractures usually occur due to one of two mechanisms: a crush injury to the digit or a sudden axial load (as in the case above).

3. A common complication that may occur with tuft fractures is a subungual hematoma. These can be treated in various ways; trephination is very effective in releasing the hematoma and reducing the pain.

4. Tuft fractures of the distal phalanx are usually stable because they are held firmly in place by surrounding normal anatomic structures. Volarly, they are secured by the fibrous network of the pulp. Distally, they are held in place by the nail plate.

Management

Because this patient has no evidence of nail bed injury, management of the fracture is simple. The patient is given a splint to prevent flexion at the DIP. The PIP is kept free. The injury is treated symptomatically with ice, and the patient is informed to return should there be later evidence of nail bed trauma. The patient should also avoid any activities that can re-injure the finger.

If there is a subungal hematoma, this will require drainage by drilling or burning a hole in the nail. This leads to rapid release of the pain and does not usually need an anesthetic.

Key points

◆   **Tuft fractures involve the distal phalanx and are usually stable injuries.**

◆   **A common associated injury is a subungual hematoma, which may require drainage.**

References

1.   Lee SG, Jupiter JB. Phalangeal and metacarpal fractures of the hand. *Hand Clin* 2000; 16(3): 323-32, vii.

2.   Hoffman DF. Management of common finger injuries. *American Family Physician*. FindArticles.com, 16 Nov. 2008.

3.   Rockwood CA, Green DP, Eds. *Fractures in Adults,* 2nd ed. Philadelphia, PA: Lippincott, 1984: 26, 317-22, 326-39, 388-94.

4.   Brunet ME, Haddad RJ Jr. Fractures and dislocations of the metacarpals and phalanges. *Clin Sports Med* 1986; 5: 773-81.

Chapter 6

Pelvis, acetabulum, hip, and femur

Case 1

Clinical presentation

A 45-year-old woman presents emergently to the trauma bay after a high-speed head-on collision. She was a restrained driver and the air bags deployed but she was noted to be unconscious at the scene. She was unable to maintain her airway and was intubated at the scene. She was hemodynamically unstable at the scene and transferred rapidly to the nearest level I trauma center. In the trauma bay, the patient remains unconscious, intubated, and hemodynamically unstable. An AP X-ray of the pelvis is taken in the trauma bay, and a STAT orthopedic consult is called.

Physical examination

On exam, the patient is intubated and sedated. You notice no gross deformities in her bilateral upper or lower extremities, no pelvic or perineal hematomas, and no open fractures. You inquire about other potential sources of bleeding. The trauma team informs you that the patient's FAST ultrasound was positive, and her chest X-ray was negative. Her rectal tone is poor secondary to the sedation that was given, but there was no blood on the exam. When you palpate her pelvis, you think it might be unstable. Neurological assessment is impossible. Based on her pelvic exam, you place a sheet around her pelvis to try and compress it.

Review the images below [Figures 1, 2 and 3]. Describe your findings.

Questions

1. What is the diagnosis?

2. What are the five joints in the pelvis?

3. What are the two classification systems for pelvic injuries and how would you classify this specific injury?

4. What do the inlet and outlet views of the pelvis help you to see?

5. When you place a pelvic sheet, where would you position it?

6. Summarize important ligaments involved with the pelvis.

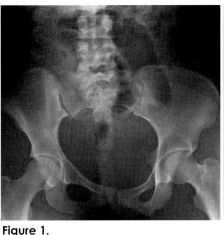

Figure 1.

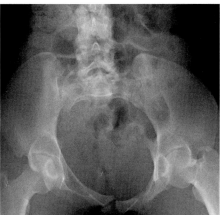

Figure 2.

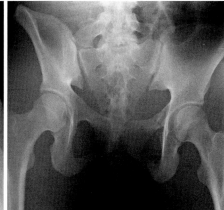

Figure 3.

Radiology findings

There is disruption of the right sacroiliac (SI) joint. The right hemipelvis is slightly displaced superiorly. There are vertical fractures involving the left superior and inferior pubic rami. The pubic symphysis is disrupted and there is a fracture through the right pubic bone.

Answers

1. Vertical shear injury of the pelvis.

2. There are five joints in the pelvis. Looking at the alignment of these five joints and knowing the mechanism of injury will all help to make a correct diagnosis. The five joints are the symphysis pubis (anteriorly), the two SI joints (posteriorly), and two hip joints. A pelvic injury always has an anterior AND a posterior component to it, never just one. Describing both components will help to identify the injury, and decide on a management strategy

3. The two classification systems for the pelvis are the Tile (AO-OTA) system, and the Young-Burgess system. The Tile system describes the pelvic injury by the degree of instability:
   i)   A: stable injury;
   ii) B: rotationally unstable;
   iii) C: both vertically and rotationally unstable.
   The Young-Burgess system divides injuries based on the mechanism and resulting deformity:
   i)   LC: lateral compression injury;
   ii) APC: anterior-posterior compression injury;
   iii) VS: vertical shear injury.
   According to the Young-Burgess classification system, this is classified as a vertical shear pelvic injury. As previously mentioned, every time there is an anterior injury, there has to be a posterior injury and vice versa. In this vertical shear injury of the pelvis, the anterior injury involves transverse fractures through both left and right pubic rami. The posterior injury involves vertical displacement through the right

SI joint. The hemipelvis is displaced cranially with complete disruption of the posterior ligaments resulting in a rotationally and vertically unstable hemipelvis, so in the Tile system this would be a C-type injury.

Vertical shear injuries occur due to a longitudinal or vertical force, such as in motor vehicle accidents, when an individual's extended leg hits the dashboard prior to impact or the driver is standing on the brake. These injuries are also seen after major falls.

4. Inlet view [Figure 2]: the X-ray beam is traditionally tilted ~45° cephalad, but recent data suggest that ~25-30° is better. On this view the pelvic brim, sacral fractures (although better visualized on the outlet view), rotational deformity of the pelvis, pubic rami fractures, widening of the pubic symphysis and SI joints can be seen. This will show posterior displacement.

   Outlet view [Figure 3]: the X-ray beam is traditionally tilted ~45° caudad, but recent data suggest that ~35° is better. This view is particularly helpful in identifying fractures in the sacral body, sacral neural foraminae, iliac wings, pubic rami, and particularly helpful for finding vertical displacement of the pelvis.

5. In placing a pelvic sheet, the landmark is the greater trochanters. The greater trochanters are palpated, and the sheet is wrapped so that it lies over the top of them, thus compressing the pelvis.

6. Pelvic trauma can include major bony fractures and disruption of ligaments. Below is a simplified list of how to think of these ligaments:
   i)   sacrotuberous ligament: attaches from the ischial tuberosity to the sacrum (prevents rotational deformity of the hemipelvis);
   ii) sacrospinous ligament: attaches from the ischial spine to the sacrum (prevents rotational deformity of the pelvis);
   iii) anterior SI ligaments: attach from the anterior sacral cortex to the ilium (prevent vertical deformity of the pelvis);

iv) posterior SI ligaments: attach from the iliac tuberosity to the sacral cortex and fifth lumbar vertebrae to the iliac crest (prevent vertical deformity of the pelvis);

v) iliolumbar ligaments: attach from the posterior pelvis to the tip of the L5 transverse process.

Management

In parallel with general resuscitation and transfusion the initial application of a wrap around sheet around the trochanters and knees will provide some control of a pelvic fracture. If there is vertical displacement, traction via a distal femoral pin on the affected side will also help. Definitive, specialist operative stabilization will be required.

This patient has a positive FAST ultrasound, is unstable, and will go directly to the operating theater for an exploratory laparotomy. The orthopedic surgeon must also be there so the operative management can be co-ordinated, as bleeding and hypotension may be due to the pelvic injury. The patient should be placed supine on a radiolucent operating table and access to the whole pelvis confirmed. In this case the general surgeon will start with the laparotomy. Initial application of an external fixator and traction may be useful and with transfusion may control the hypotension. Persisting hypotension may require formal pelvic stabilization or angiographic embolization.

The anterior pelvis can be stabilized with external or internal fixation depending on the anterior fracture pattern. The posterior pelvis is usually stabilized percutaneously with the placement of iliosacral screws. This is a specialist procedure but temporary anterior external fixation and the application of longitudinal traction should help control the situation and be available anywhere.

Key points

- Vertical shear injuries result from high-energy vertical forces and produce an unstable pelvic ring. Patients can bleed to death.

- Vertical shear injuries are associated with other serious traumatic injuries involving multiple local and distant organs and structures.

- Unstable pelvic fractures are a frequent source of major bleeding. Other sites include the chest, peritoneum, other retroperitoneal sites, the long bones and external hemorrhage. In this scenario, the chest X-ray was negative and there was no external blood loss or long bone injury. With a positive FAST this patient may have a significant abdominal injury and needs a laparotomy in association with control of any pelvic bleeding.

- Mechanical stabilization of the pelvis with a sheet either at the scene or in the ER is often very helpful and may control local bleeding. The sheet should be replaced early by definitive fixation.

References

1. Burgess AR, Eastridge BJ, Young JW, *et al.* Pelvic ring disruptions: effective classification system and treatment protocols. *J Trauma* 1990; 30(7): 848-56.

2. Young JW, Burgess AR, Brumback RJ, Poka A. Pelvic fractures: value of plain radiography in early assessment and management. *Radiology* 1986; 160(2): 445-51.

3. Bucholz RW, Heckman JD, Court-Brown CM, *et al*, Eds. *Rockwood and Green's Fractures in Adults*, 6th ed. Philadelphia, PA: Lippincott Williams & Wilkins, 2006.

Case 2

Clinical presentation

A 37-year-old male presents to the ER after a high-speed motor vehicle accident. He is unconscious and hemodynamically stable at the scene. He was intubated at the scene, and presents to the ER still hemodynamically unstable. AP pelvic X-rays are obtained and shown below. A FAST ultrasound is positive. The patient is rushed to the operating theater. The trauma workup thus far has shown pelvic and abdominal injuries.

Physical examination

On gross physical exam, it is noted that the patient's leg lengths are equal. There is no deformity of the bilateral lower extremities. There is no blood at the urethral meatus, and there is no blood on rectal exam. The patient's rectal tone is weak, but he has also been given sedatives for his intubation. His pelvis is palpated and is noted to be grossly unstable,

especially with internal and external rotation. A sheet is immediately placed around his pelvis for compression.

Review the image below [Figure 4]. Describe your findings.

Questions

1. What is the diagnosis?

2. What is the mechanism of injury?

3. How is this injury classified?

4. What are the four major sources of bleeding in a polytrauma patient?

5. How can the elastic recoil of the pelvis affect the decision making process?

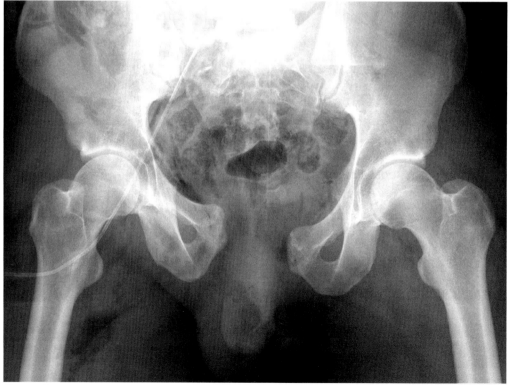

Figure 4.

Radiology findings

A single frontal view of the pelvis demonstrates diastasis of the symphysis pubis measuring approximately 5.2cm. There is also a comminuted fracture of the right sacral ala (resulting in disrupted neural arches). Both hip joints are well maintained. The pubic rami are unremarkable bilaterally. The SI joints are grossly intact. There is also vertical malalignment of the pubic bones.

Answers

1. Unstable anterior posterior compression (APC III, or 'C' type) injury of the pelvis ('open book pelvis').

2. An anteroposterior force is applied to the pelvis. This force acts as a lever arm on one side of the pelvis, pulling it out, thus opening it up like the pages in a book. This pelvis is very unstable, especially on physical exam to internal and external rotation. Hence, the name 'open book pelvis'.

3. For a discussion on the Tile classification system, and the Young-Burgess classification system, please see the earlier discussion on the vertical shear pelvic injury (p114).

    For this particular fracture, based on the Young-Burgess classfication system, this is an APC III injury. To understand pelvic injuries it is important to remember that the pelvis is a ring with an anterior and posterior component. Both need to break in a displaced injury:
    i)   APC I: lower-energy injury. Anterior component: <2cm of widening of the pubic symphysis. Posterior component: little to no widening of the SI joint;
    ii) APC II: higher-energy injury. Anterior component: >2cm of widening of the pubic symphysis or widened pubic ramii fractures. Posterior component: widening of the anterior portion of the SI joint, disruption of the sacrotuberous ligament,

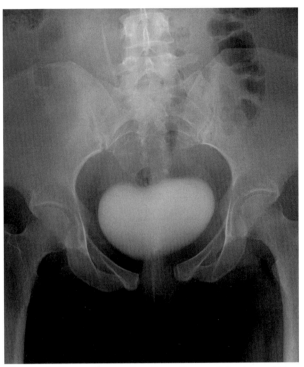

Figure 5. There is greater than 2cm widening of the pubic symphysis, but it is unclear if there is disruption posteriorly at the SI joint. However, if correlated with physical exam and there is rotational instability, this can be considered an APC II injury.

sacrospinous ligament, and muscles of the pelvic floor. This cannot be seen on plain radiographs; however, these ligamentous and pelvic injuries contribute to the rotational instability of the pelvis that is felt on physical exam [Figure 5];
iii) APC III: higher-energy, continuous force. Anterior component: widening of the pubic symphysis or pubic ramii fractures. Posterior component: complete tearing of the posterior SI ligaments, allowing the ilium to displace from the sacrum posteriorly. These injuries are rotationally and vertically unstable. There is a very high mortality rate with these injuries [Figure 6].

4. The four major sources of bleeding in a poly-trauma patient include the chest, peritoneum, retroperitoneum, and long bones. In any hemodynamically unstable trauma patient, these

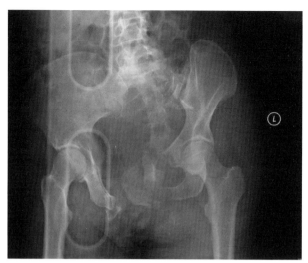

Figure 6. There are comminuted fractures involving both the superior and inferior pubic rami bilaterally. There is marked displacement of the pubic bones towards the right of the midline. There is disruption of the left sacroiliac joint. There is a comminuted fracture of the left sacral ala. The posterior damage makes this an APC III injury. To further define the injury type, a CT scan is indicated to examine the posterior structures.

additional areas should be assessed. APC injuries have a very high risk of major bleeding.

5. The pelvis has elastic recoil, and even after severe deformation, it can sometimes recoil to near normal alignment. This can be confusing for the clinician because the severity on physical exam does not match the lack of severity on imaging. The image may not show the correct extent of the injury, but the physical exam should guide the physician as to the true nature of pelvic trauma. If a sheet is applied, the fracture may also appear fully reduced and the degree of injury be under appreciated.

Management

In this case, in the immediate unstable situation, a sheet should be placed around the greater trochanters to compress the pelvis. The patient can

then be taken to the operating theater where a variety of procedures may be performed according to the experience of the surgeon. These range from application of an external fixator to 'close the book' or direct operative stabilization. A full description of these is beyond the remit of this book. In addition to the potential for major hemorrhage, severe pelvic fractures are associated with abdominal trauma, genitourinary trauma and remote injury. Each may also require definitive management. Definitive stabilization of the pelvis involves plating of the pubis through a Pfannenstiel or vertical incision and stabilization of the posterior ring either with an anterior sacroiliac plate or with iliosacral screws passed under X-ray control. These are procedures for experienced pelvic surgeons.

In general, APC I injuries can be treated non-operatively while APC II fractures usually only require anterior fixation. APC III injuries require both anterior and posterior fixation.

Key points

♦ Anterior-posterior compression injuries can usually be diagnosed based on knowing the mechanism of injury and on physical exam. Open book pelvic injures are APC injuries.

♦ There are three types of APC injuries associated with worsening degrees of pelvic instability.

♦ Initial stabilization of an unstable pelvis involves placement of a pelvic sheet and often initial stabilization of the pelvis with an external fixator.

♦ In addition to the pelvis, it is essential to examine the hemodynamically unstable patient for additional sources of bleeding elsewhere, even if at the time of presentation the pelvis appears to be the most obvious source.

References

1. Kam J, Jackson H, Ben-Menachem Y. Vascular injuries in blunt pelvic trauma. *Radiol Clin North Am* 1981; 19: 171-86.

2. Bucholz RW, Heckman JD, Court-Brown CM, *et al*, Eds. *Rockwood and Green's Fractures in Adults*, 6th ed. Philadelphia, PA: Lippincott Williams & Wilkins, 2006.

3. Tile M, Ed. *Fractures of the Pelvis and Acetabulum*, 2nd ed. Baltimore, MD: Williams & Wilkins, 1995: 41-52.

4. Gibbs MA, Bosse MJ. Pelvic ring fractures. In: *Trauma Management: An Emergency Medicine Approach*. Ferrera PC, Colucciello SA, Marx JA, Verdile VP, Gibbs MA, Eds. St Louis, MO: Mosby, 1998: 330-3.

5. Green DP, Ed. *Fractures in Adults*, 2nd ed. Philadelphia, PA: Lippincott, 1984.

6. Junkins EP, Nelson DS, Carroll KL, Hansen K, Furnival RA. A prospective evaluation of the clinical presentation of pediatric pelvic fractures. *J Trauma* 2001; 51: 64-8.

7. Failinger MS, McGanity PLJ. Unstable fractures of the pelvic ring. *J Bone Joint Surg [Am]* 1992; 745: 781-91.

8. Guyton JL, Crockarell JR Jr. Fractures of acetabulum and pelvis. In: *Campbell's Operative Orthopedics*, 10th ed. Canale ST, Ed. St Louis, MO: Mosby, 2003: 2939-84.

Case 3

Clinical presentation

A 62-year-old woman falls from a step stool while reaching up to grab something from a cabinet. She lands on her side and complains of pain in her hips immediately afterwards, and has difficulty rising. She is brought to the ER for evaluation. She did not hit her head, she is currently hemodynamically stable, and she is only complaining of bilateral hip pain. Pelvic images are obtained, and an orthopedic consult is called.

Physical examination

The patient has equal leg lengths, both legs are easily internally and externally rotated, but this causes pain in the hip, worse on the right. The pelvis feels stable to internal and external rotation, as well as to posterior compression. The patient complains of pain when her pelvis is manipulated. Otherwise, she has good rectal tone, with no blood noted on rectal exam, no blood at the urethra and intact perineal skin. Distally, she has no neurovascular deficits.

Review the image below [Figure 7]. Describe your findings.

Questions

1. What is the diagnosis?

2. What is the mechanism of injury?

3. What are some of the lines that can be used on an AP X-ray of the pelvis to help identify a subtle pelvic injury?

4. Describe findings that can indicate an open pelvis.

5. What are the standard surgical approaches to the anterior and posterior pelvis?

6. Describe the injuries that occur in an LC II and LC III pelvis.

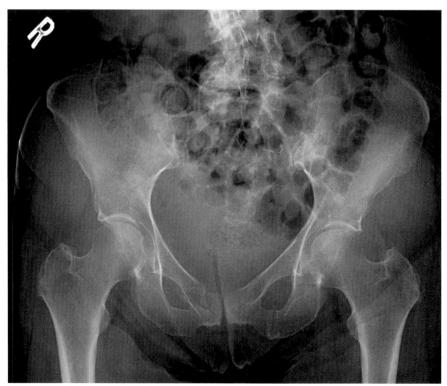

Figure 7.

Radiology findings

There are acute fractures of the superior and inferior right pubic ramii. There is no obvious widening of the SI joints bilaterally.

Answers

1. Lateral compression (LC I) pelvic injury.

2. The LC I pelvic injury is the most common type of pelvic fracture. It is caused by a lateral compression applied to the hemipelvis. It is a stable injury with no mechanical instability in any plane.

3. To identify pelvic fractures it is helpful to look at the iliopectineal line: a line drawn from the ilium to just above the superior pubic ramus to join with the pubic symphysis. It is primarily used for assessment of acetabular fractures but disruption will be seen in anterior pelvic ring (superior pubic ramus) fractures. The ilioischial line connects the ilium with the ischium and is used to assess stability of the posterior column. The best line to assess posteriorly on an AP X-ray is the continuation of the internal brim of the pelvis on to the sacrum. It should line up with the arch of the second sacral foramina. The sacral foramina in general are an important feature to assess as any compression of the sacrum often occurs through this area (sacral zone 2) and distortion of the foramina may be seen.

4. Signs of an open pelvic injury include: open wounds around the pelvis or perineum, or bleeding into the rectum or vagina.

5. Anterior pelvis: Pfannenstiel or Stoppa approaches. Posterior pelvis: iliac approach to the iliac fossa and SI joint, or the formal direct posterior approach to the sacrum.

6. LC II and III injuries are much more severe injuries. They are due to high-energy trauma to the pelvis. They are often found after major falls, crushing injuries or in side impact motor vehicle crashes.

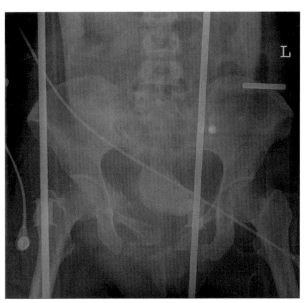

Figure 8. LC II pelvic fracture. There is a fracture of the right superior and inferior pubic ramus, with widening of the right SI joint. There is contrast in the bladder.

In the LC II [Figure 8] pelvic fracture, there are complete anterior and posterior injuries. The pelvis is rotationally unstable but vertically stable. In the LC III pelvic fracture, the LC II fracture on one side is accompanied by an AP II fracture on the opposite side as the force has continued across the whole pelvis. This injury has been termed a 'windswept pelvis.'

Management

LC I injuries can be managed non-operatively since they are stable injuries. The patient can weight bear as tolerated, with adequate pain control. LC II and III injuries require operative fixation. For these injures, there is debate over whether or not a sheet placed in the ER is helpful, because they are already volume decreasing injuries so applying a compression device will only increase the deformity. It is unlikely there will be any harm caused by sheeting. LC fractures are not associated with the same volume of massive pelvic hemorrhage as seen in high-grade AP or VS injuries. They are more often a marker of the application of major force to the patient and an indication to assess elsewhere for major bleeding.

Definitively, an LC II injury requires surgical stabilization with both anterior and posterior stabilization. Anteriorly, an external fixator is commonly used if the anterior lesion is a ramus fracture. Posterior stabilization depends on the experience of the surgeon but it is common practise to insert iliosacral screws. Often, patients with major pelvic injuries are allowed minimal weight bearing on the side of the unstable posterior injury for three months.

Key points

♦ LC I pelvic fractures are the most common type of pelvic injury.

♦ LC I injuries are usually managed non-operatively, as they are vertically and rotationally stable fractures.

♦ LC II pelvic injuries have an unstable hemipelvis in compression. These injuries require operative stabilization.

♦ LC III injuries, also called a windswept pelvis, are usually high-energy injuries with unstable patients, and usually require emergent fixation with a pelvic external fixator, and definitive fixation when possible.

References

1. Lunsjo K, Tadros A, Hauggaard A, Blomgren R, Kopke J, Abu-Zidan FM. Associated injuries and not fracture instability predict mortality in pelvic fractures: a prospective study of 100 patients. *J Trauma* 2007; 62(3): 687-91

2. Bucholz RW, Heckman JD, Court-Brown CM, *et al*, Eds. *Rockwood and Green's Fractures in Adults*, 6th ed. Philadelphia, PA: Lippincott Williams & Wilkins, 2006.

3. Holdsworth FW. Dislocation and fracture-dislocation of the pelvis. *J Bone and Joint Surg [Am]* 1948; 30B: 461-6.

4. Tile M. Acute pelvic fractures: I. Causation and classification. *J Am Acad Orthop Surg* 1996; 4(3): 143-51.

5. Hanson R, Milne J, Chapman M. Open fractures of the pelvis: review of 43 cases. *J Bone Joint Surg* 1991; 73: 325-9.

6. Tile M. Acute pelvic fractures: II. Principles of management. *J Am Acad Orthop Surg* 1996; 4(3): 152-61.

7. Richardson JD, Hardy J, Amin MM, Flint LM. Open pelvic fractures. *J Trauma* 1982; 22: 533-8.

8. Burgess AR, Eastridge BJ, Young JW. Pelvic ring disruptions: effective classification system and treatment protocols. *J Trauma* 1990; 30(7): 848-56

Case 4

Clinical presentation

A 61-year-old man is involved in a high-speed motor vehicle accident. He has a GCS of 15 and is hemodynamically stable at the scene and in the trauma bay. His trauma workup thus far reveals a low-grade splenic laceration. He is complaining of right hip pain and an orthopedic evaluation is performed in the trauma bay.

Physical examination

The patient is lying supine on the bed. Grossly, no leg length discrepancies are noted. There is no internal/external rotation of one hip compared with another. There are minor abrasions over the right knee with an effusion. The patient has pain on log-roll of the right hip. Assessment of range of motion is not possible secondary to pain. There appears to be some swelling over the hemipelvis. Distally, the patient is able to plantarflex and dorsiflex his foot without difficulty. He has palpable popliteal, posterior tibia, and dorsalis pedis pulses.

Review the image below [Figure 9]. Describe your findings.

Questions

1. What is the diagnosis?

2. What is the mechanism of injury?

3. What is the goal of treating acetabular fractures?

4. What additional X-rays are needed to correctly diagnose this fracture?

5. How are these fractures classified?

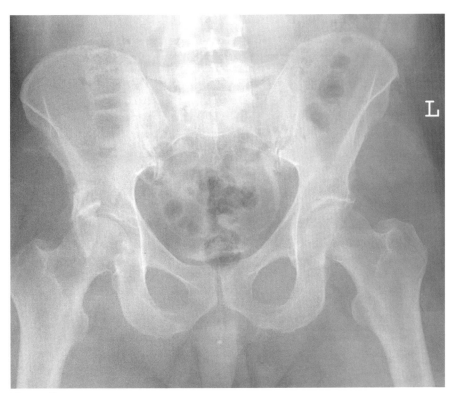

Figure 9.

Radiology findings

There is a fracture of the posterior wall of the right acetabulum, with multiple fragments posteriorly, possibly in the joint space.

Answers

1.   Posterior wall fracture of the acetabulum.

2.   The mechanism of injury is by an axial load applied to the distal femur, which is transmitted up the shaft and through the hip joint to the acetabulum. The amount of displacement of fracture fragments and the fracture pattern depends on the position of the hip at the time of impact, the amount of force, and the quality of bone.

3.   The goal of treating acetabular fractures is to salvage a longlasting stable hip joint. This is achieved by obtaining and maintaining an anatomic congruent reduction of the articular surface and a stable hip joint.

4.   In addition to the AP X-ray of the pelvis in the trauma bay, two Judet views are also needed. These are the iliac oblique and the obturator oblique views which define the columns and walls of the acetabulum. A CT scan is also required to fully define the fracture pattern. If there is an associated pelvic injury, inlet and outlet views of the pelvis should also be obtained. Each radiographic view provides identification of specific lines and anatomical landmarks that help define the fracture classification. When viewing AP pelvis, obturator oblique and iliac oblique films, different aspects of the pelvis are best visualized, as below:
     i)   AP pelvis: defines the iliopectineal line, the ilioischial line, the posterior rim of the acetabulum, the anterior rim of the acetabulum, the teardrop, and the sourcil. The iliopectineal line marks the anterior column of the acetabulum. The ilioischial line

marks the posterior column of the acetabulum. The sourcil (French for eyebrow, and looks like an eyebrow on X-ray) is the roof of the acetabulum. The posterior rim represents the posterior wall and the anterior rim represents the anterior wall. The teardrop is the fovea;
     ii)   obturator oblique: allows visualization of the anterior column and posterior wall. This X-ray is taken with the beam angled 45° towards the obturator foramen; hence, the obturator foramen is seen on this view;
     iii) iliac oblique: allows visualization of the posterior column and anterior wall. The X-ray beam is angled at 45° to the ilium. The iliac wing is seen on this view.
     The ilium and the obturator foramen are at 90° to each other, therefore, an iliac oblique view of one side, is also an obturator oblique view of the contralateral side. For example, an iliac oblique view of the right acetabulum will give an obturator oblique view of the left acetabulum, and vice versa.

5.   The Letournel and Judet classification divides acetabular fractures into five simple and five complex types:
     i)   simple types: anterior column, anterior wall, posterior column, posterior wall, and transverse fractures;
     ii)   complex types: transverse and posterior wall, posterior column and posterior wall, T-type, anterior column/posterior hemi-transverse and associated both column fractures.
     Posterior wall fractures [Figures 10 and 11] are the most common type of acetabular fracture and are seen on both AP and obturator oblique views. On X-ray, the posterior rim will be disrupted in two locations, representing a free fragment. It is important to look for loose bony fragments in the joint, an amount of disruption of the articular surface, and any associated femoral head fractures that occur as the force is transmitted through the femur. These will be best seen on the CT scan.

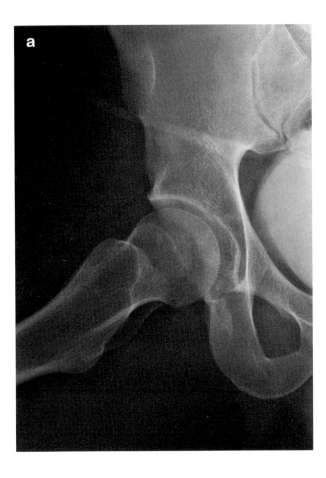

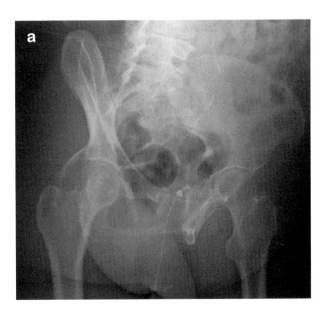

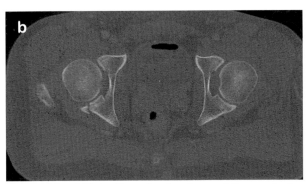

Figure 10. a) Plain film of a fracture of the posterior acetabular wall in this 23-year-old male. b) The injury is better depicted on axial CT.

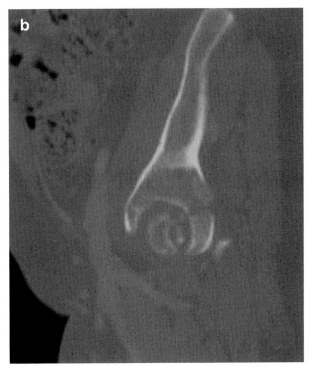

Figure 11. a) A Judet view in this 60-year-old female allows for better appreciation of a fracture of the posterior wall of the acetabulum. b) However, a sagittal CT image best depicts the fracture.

Transverse fractures [Figure 12] are considered elementary fractures; however, the fracture crosses both the anterior and posterior columns. Because both columns are disrupted in this fracture, disruption of the iliopectineal and ilioischial lines are seen on the AP X-ray of the pelvis. The articular surface is also involved, so there is disruption of the anterior and posterior acetabular rims.

Associated both column fractures [Figure 13] are the most common complex fracture. In this fracture pattern, both the anterior and posterior column are vertically split from each other and transversely separated from the rest of the pelvis so that no articular surface is connected to the axial skeleton. The both column fracture is unique in that it may display secondary congruence. Secondary congruence is where, despite fractures involving the articular surface, it remains well aligned to the femoral head due to displacement of both anterior and posterior columns around the femoral head as it medializes during fracture. A spur sign, seen on the obturator oblique view, is also diagnostic of a both column fracture.

Management

The decision to operate on an acetabular fracture depends on numerous factors, such as the age of the patient, pre-injury level of function, and associated medical comorbidities. Aside from patient factors, fracture factors are also considered in the equation. These include the degree of articular displacement, the position of any intact segments and associated features such as marginal impaction or intra-articular free fragments. Adequacy of the roof segment can be measured by the roof arcs and, if adequate, non-operative management can be considered. The roof arc is measured by drawing a vertical line through the center of the femoral head on an AP view. A second line is then drawn connecting the center of the femoral head to the edge of the remaining articular surface. If the angle between these two lines is >45°, then the weight bearing dome is adequate, and there is a decreased chance of the patient experiencing post-traumatic arthritis/hip instability. Roof arc measurements are not applicable for posterior wall fractures; here the decision depends on the stability of the hip joint and the amount of wall involved. If the hip

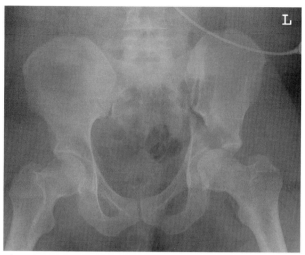

Figure 12. Transverse fracture of the left acetabulum. There is disruption of the sourcil, iliopectineal line and ilioischial line.

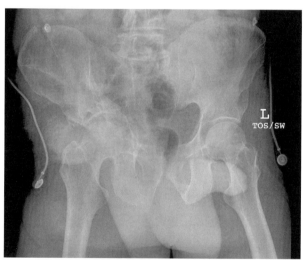

Figure 13. Both column fracture of the right acetabulum. Multiple fractures are noted involving the right hemipelvis. The iliac wing is fractured, and there is disruption of the iliopectineal and ilioischial lines, and the superior and inferior pubic rami. Essentially the whole acetabulum is driven medially.

can easily dislocate, surgical fixation of the posterior wall is necessary. This is usually seen with >40% of posterior wall involvement. Therefore, <40% of posterior wall involvement may be a consideration for non-operative intervention. Most both column fractures are inherently unstable and will require fixation. However, if secondary congruence is noted on all three X-rays (ilioinguinal, obturator oblique, and AP), non-operative treatment can be considered.

Often, however, these injuries heal poorly with the affected extremity shortened and medialized.

The goal of surgery is to appropriately align the articular surface to prevent an unstable and arthritic hip, and allow return to pre-injury level of function. The surgical approach is chosen based on the classification and displacement of the fracture. The Kocher-Langenbeck approach is usually used for posterior wall and column fractures. The ilioinguinal approach is usually used for anterior column and wall fractures. An extended iliofemoral approach can allow access to both the anterior and posterior acetabulum.

A full discussion of acetabular fractures is beyond the remit of this text - readers are thus referred to Letournel's textbook (see reference 2).

Key points

- Acetabular fractures are rarely life-threatening injuries. Their surgical treatment is much easier if done within the first few days but special experience and adequate planning is necessary. The appropriate images and studies should be obtained prior to fixation.

- Based on the Letournel and Judet classification, there are ten types of acetabular fractures: five simple types and five complex fractures.

- The obturator oblique view allows visualization of the anterior column and posterior wall. The iliac oblique view allows visualization of the posterior column and anterior wall.

- The six lines seen on acetabular X-rays are the ilioischial (posterior column), iliopectineal (anterior column), posterior rim (posterior wall), anterior rim (anterior wall), sourcil (weight bearing dome), and the teardrop lines (medial confluence).

- Operative indications include articular displacement >2mm, roof arc >45°, >40% of posterior wall involvement, and femoral head subluxation.

References

1. Bucholz RW, Heckman JD, Court-Brown CM, *et al*, Eds. *Rockwood and Green's Fractures in Adults*, 6th ed. Philadelphia, PA: Lippincott Williams & Wilkins, 2006.

2. Letournel E. *Fractures of the Acetabulum*, 2nd ed. New York, NY: Springer-Verlag, 1993.

3. Dakin GJ, Eberhardt AW, Alonso JE, *et al*. Acetabular fracture patterns: associations with motor vehicle crash information. *J Trauma* 1999; 47(6): 1063-71.

4. Judet R, Judet J, Letournel E. Fractures of the acetabulum: classification and surgical approaches for open reduction. Preliminary report. *J Bone Joint Surg [Am]* 1964; 46: 1615-46.

5. Olson SA. CT-based acetabular fracture classification. *AJR Am J Roentgenol* 2005; 185(1): 277-8; author reply 278-80.

6. Beaulé PE, Dorey FJ, Matta JM. Letournel classification for acetabular fractures. Assessment of interobserver and intraobserver reliability. *J Bone Joint Surg [Am]* 2003; 85-A(9): 1704-9.

7. Tile M. *Fractures of the Pelvis and Acetabulum*, 2nd ed. Baltimore, MD: Williams & Wilkins, 1995.

Case 5

Clinical presentation

A 36-year-old man presents to the ER after a high-speed motor vehicle accident. He was a restrained driver, and the airbags deployed. He was alert and oriented at the scene, and complaining of right hip pain. In the trauma bay he remains alert and oriented, hemodynamically stable, and continues to complain of right hip pain. A complete trauma workup including an AP pelvic X-ray is performed, the patient is taken for a CT scan, and an orthopedic consult is called based on the results of the CT scan seen below.

Physical examination

At first glance, the patient's right leg appears shorter than the left leg. The right leg is externally rotated and abducted. He has pain and resists any attempted range of motion of his right hip. Distally there is a palpable dorsalis pedis and posterior tibial pulse, and he is able to move his foot and toes normally, although he is uncomfortable during the exam. He has good sensation in the L4/L5/S1 distributions.

Review the images below [Figures 14 and 15]. Describe your findings.

Questions

1. What is the diagnosis?

2. What is the mechanism of injury?

3. How are these injuries classified?

4. Without a CT scan, how can this injury be diagnosed?

5. What other injuries may occur?

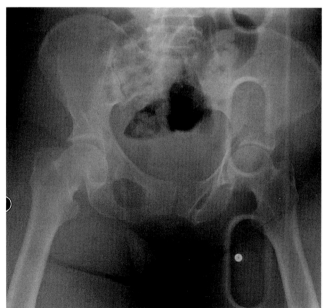

Figure 14.

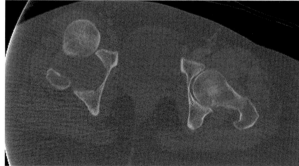

Figure 15.

Radiology findings

An AP view of the pelvis demonstrates that the right hip is not congruent. The joint space is widened, compared with the normal left side. The femur is externally rotated and the lesser trochanter is prominent. There are no fractures of the femoral head or acetabulum, further confirmed with a CT scan (seen above). It is occasionally difficult to distinguish an anterior hip dislocation from a posterior hip dislocation. In an anterior dislocation, the lesser trochanter is prominent and the femur is externally rotated. In a posterior dislocation, the lesser trochanter is less prominent and the femur is typically internally rotated.

Answers

1. Anterior hip dislocation.

2. Anterior hip dislocations are usually due to a high-energy trauma, and occur due to forced abduction and external rotation of the hip joint. These injuries can be seen in a fall from height, or in a motor vehicle accident (the abducted hip joint strikes the dashboard).

3. Hip dislocations are divided into three groups: anterior, posterior (most common) and central. In anterior dislocations, the femoral head is displaced into the obturator, pubic or iliac region. In posterior dislocations, the femoral head lies lateral and superior to the acetabulum and the femur is adducted and internally rotated. In central dislocations, the femoral head projects into the pelvis and there is always an associated acetabular fracture.

4. Anterior hip dislocations are often difficult to diagnose with an AP pelvic X-ray only. However, in the trauma bay this is often the only image, aside from a chest X-ray, that is possible to obtain. Clues to help on the AP pelvis are that with an anterior dislocation, the femoral head on the dislocated hip can appear larger than the non-dislocated hip because it is closer to the X-ray source. The joint space may not be congruent or differ in width from the normal side. The physical exam aids in making the diagnosis, and when able, a lateral X-ray of the suspected hip can radiographically confirm the diagnosis.

5. Anterior dislocations of the hip can be associated with femoral head, acetabular, greater trochanter, femoral neck and femoral shaft fractures (better diagnosed on CT imaging). Avulsion fractures of the anterior inferior iliac spine (AIIS) may also occur. There may be concomitant injury to the femoral artery, femoral vein, or femoral nerve.

Management

The patient can be consciously sedated in the ER, and a closed reduction should be attempted. The patient is placed supine on the table. The assistant should hold down the pelvis, while the surgeon applies axial traction while internally and externally rotating the hip. This will dislodge it from the superior lip of the acetabulum. The hip should then reduce. The assistant may push down on the femoral head to help push it back into the acetabulum.

Indications for open reduction in the operating theater include the inability to close reduce, or an associated acetabular or femoral neck/head fracture.

Key points

- Anterior hip dislocations are often difficult to diagnose, and a lateral X-ray of the hip or CT scan may be required to confirm suspicions based on physical exam.
- To reduce the hip, axial traction is applied with simultaneous internal and external rotation of the femoral head.
- Indications for open reduction in the operating theater include the inability to close reduce, or an associated femoral head/neck fracture.

References

1. Koval KJ, Zuckerman JD. *Handbook of Fractures*, 3rd ed. Philadelphia, PA: Lippincott Williams & Wilkins, 2006.
2. Bucholz RW, Heckman JD, Court-Brown CM, *et al*. *Rockwood and Green's Fractures in Adults*, 6th ed. Philadelphia, PA: Lippincott Williams & Wilkins, 2006.

Case 6

Clinical presentation

A 36-year-old man presents to the ER after a high-speed motor vehicle accident. He was a restrained driver, and the airbags deployed. He was intubated at the scene for trouble maintaining his airway. He was hemodynamically stable at the scene. While in the trauma bay, he remains intubated and hemodynamically stable. A complete trauma workup is performed, and an orthopedic consult is called based on the results of the AP pelvic X-ray below.

Physical examination

The patient is intubated and sedated. It is noted that his right leg is held in external rotation, abduction, and slight flexion. There is no gross deformity of the knee and thigh, and although they appear structurally intact, the leg is held in a fixed abnormal position and any attempt to move the hip meets significant resistance. Motor and sensory exam are altered by sedation. However, distally, a downgoing Babinski's reflex and normal pulses are noted.

Review the image below [Figure 16]. Describe your findings.

Questions

1. What is the diagnosis?

2. What is the mechanism of injury?

3. What other injuries may occur?

4. Before reduction, what additional injury should you look for?

5. Why is it so important to reduce the dislocation as soon as possible?

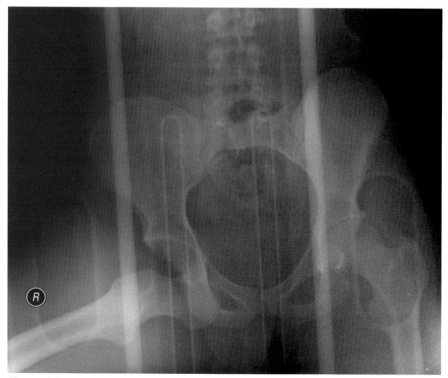

Figure 16.

Radiology findings

On an AP view of the pelvis, the right femoral head is displaced anteriorly and inferiorly relative to the acetabulum and overlies the obturator foramen. The extremity is held in external rotation, and abduction. There may be an impaction fracture on the femoral head but no other obvious fractures are identified.

Answers

1. Anterior hip dislocation (inferior obturator type).

2. Anterior hip dislocations usually occur in high-energy trauma, as the impact hits an externally rotated, abducted, and flexed hip. The hip dislocates inferiorly in this position.

3. The inferior type of anterior hip dislocation is associated with impaction (indentation) fractures of the femoral head. These occur after impaction of the femoral head against the anteroinferior rim of the acetabulum. Hence, these injuries are located at the superolateral aspect of the femoral head. They are similar to a Hill-Sachs deformity in the shoulder and often appear as a depressed fracture or flattening of the femoral head. Neurovascular injuries are not common with anterior inferior hip dislocations; however, they can occur and should be examined for. These injuries are high-energy injuries, and additional orthopedic trauma to the ipsilateral extremity should be examined for, such as fractures of the acetabulum, pelvis, or femur. Spine injuries are also associated. Non-orthopedic trauma injuries, such as blunt abdominal injuries, or chest injuries such as fractured ribs and a pneumothorax, should also be sought as part of a full trauma assessment.

4. Femoral neck fracture. If a femoral neck fracture is present, then a closed reduction in the ER should not be attempted. The patient needs to go to the operating theater.

5. The blood supply to the femoral head is at risk in any hip dislocation. To decrease the risk of osteonecrosis, the hip should be reduced without delay. The main blood supply to the femoral head is from the medial femoral circumflex artery through branches that travel along the surface of the posterior neck within the capsule. They are at risk in any dislocation or femoral neck fracture.

Management

An initial closed reduction should be attempted in the ER under conscious sedation. For anteriorly dislocated hips, an effective method of reduction is to lie the patient supine on the table. The assistant should hold the pelvis. The surgeon should then apply longitudinal traction while gently internally and externally rotating the hip. This will dislodge the hip from the inferior lip of the acetabulum. Once free, the joint should automatically want to relocate. The assistant can also apply upward pressure on the femoral head to coax it into the acetabulum. For anterior dislocations, if a reduction is successful, there is no need for an abduction pillow. The patient should be kept in a position of adduction and internal rotation to prevent re-dislocaton; this can be done with a brace. The patient, when able, can then partial weight bear, and progress to weight bearing as tolerated over a period of three weeks. Indications for open reduction in the operating theater include the inability to obtain a closed reduction, associated acetabular or femoral head/neck fractures or an unstable hip joint that easily re-dislocates after closed reduction.

Surgically an anterior dislocation is usually approached via an anterior Smith-Peterson approach or the anterolateral Watson-Jones approach. A lateral Hardinge approach can also be used but allows less access to the femoral head.

Key points

- Anterior hip dislocations are usually the result of high-energy trauma, and associated injuries should be sought.

- Longitudinal traction with internal and external rotation of the femoral head is an effective means of reduction.

- The major blood supply to the femoral head is at risk in dislocation, and arises from the medial and lateral femoral circumflex arteries which branch off the profunda femoris.

- For anterior-inferior hip dislocations, the patient's extremity is found to be abducted, markedly externally rotated, with flexion.

References

1. Campbell WC. *Campbell's Operative Orthopaedics*, Vol. III, 9th ed. St Louis, MO: CX Mosby Co: 2232-4.

2. Epstein HC, Wiss DA. Traumatic anterior dislocation of the hip. *Orthopaedics* 1985; 8: 132-4.

3. Bucholz RW, Heckman JD, Court-Brown CM, *et al. Rockwood and Green's Fractures in Adults*, 6th ed. Philadelphia, PA: Lippincott Williams & Wilkins, 2006.

Case 7

Clinical presentation

A 27-year-old female front-seat passenger presents to the ER after a high-speed motor vehicle accident. She was intubated at the scene, and is hemodynamically stable. She presents to the trauma bay intubated, and is hemodynamically stable. The trauma team notices an obvious deformity of her right leg. An AP pelvic X-ray is obtained, and an orthopedic consult is called.

Physical examination

On exam, the patient is intubated and sedated. Her right leg is shortened, adducted, and internally rotated with some flexion. No abnormality of the knee is noticed, and a range of motion of the knee is possible without difficulty. There is difficulty with range of motion of the hip, especially with external rotation and hip extension. Distally, there are palpable dorsalis pedis and tibial pulses, as well as a down-going Babinski's reflex. Further motor exam will not be useful until the patient is able to follow commands.

Review the image below [Figure 17]. Describe your findings.

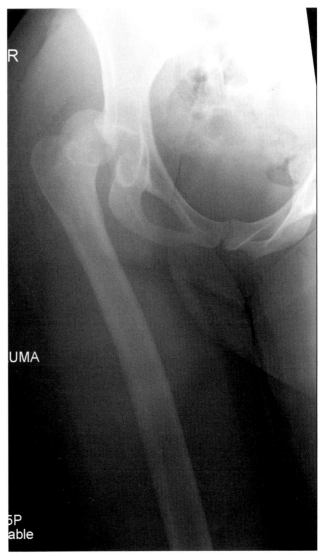

Figure 17.

Questions

1. What is the diagnosis?

2. What is the mechanism of injury?

3. What other injuries might be present?

4. List long-term complications that may occur from this injury.

5. How are these injuries classified?

6. On plain films, how would you determine whether a hip dislocation is anterior or posterior?

Radiology findings

There is a posterior dislocation of the right hip. The right femoral head is displaced posteriorly and superiorly and it overlaps the roof of the acetabulum. The proximal femur is internally rotated, shown by a reduced profile of the lesser trochanter. There are no associated fractures of the acetabulum or femoral head; this is confirmed on CT imaging [Figure 18]. CT imaging is a valuable imaging modality used to determine the presence of associated fractures and small intra-articular fracture fragments.

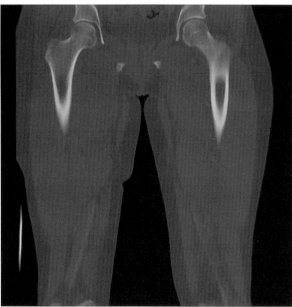

Figure 18. Coronal CT image of the bilateral hip joints after reduction demonstrates no fractures, no loose bodies, and a congruent reduction.

Answers

1. Posterior hip dislocation.

2. Posterior hip dislocations in young patients are typically seen after high-energy trauma. They occur when the hip and knee are flexed, as in a seated passenger, and a force strikes the knee, driving the femur and the hip joint posteriorly. This typically occurs when there is a major frontal impact and the patient's knee strikes the dashboard. Posterior hip dislocations are more common than anterior hip dislocations.

3. There may be associated femoral head, neck or shaft fractures. Acetabular and pelvic fractures are commonly seen. Judet views are important for evaluation of the acetabulum; the posterior superior rim of the acetabulum is usually involved in posterior hip dislocations. Knee injuries, including patellar fractures, posterior knee dislocation and cruciate ligament damage, are also more frequent with posterior hip dislocations due to their common mechanism. There is a very high risk of sciatic nerve injuries as it lies just behind the hip and may be directly injured in the dislocation Other abdominal, chest and head injuries found in trauma patients should also be examined for.

4. The most common long-term complication of a hip dislocation is post-traumatic arthritis. Avascular necrosis (AVN, also known as osteonecrosis) is an important complication and can occur even with rapid reduction of the dislocated hip. Injury to the sciatic nerve may occur and usually involves the peroneal component. It is more common in posterior hip dislocations, due to the posteriorly dislocated femoral head compressing the nerve, or due to a piece of posterior superior acetabular wall fracture impinging on the nerve. Recurrent dislocation after reduction is uncommon.

5. There are a number of classification systems that have been proposed to classify hip dislocations, including the Thompson-Epstein and Pipkin schemes. However, the first basic classification is whether the dislocation is anterior or posterior. Brumback *et al* proposed a classification system which incorporates both anterior and posterior classifications and associated fractures. Perhaps the most important distinction to make is the direction of the dislocation and associated injuries.

6. Clinical examination should clarify whether a dislocation is anterior or posterior as the position of the leg is characteristic. On plain films the deformity is also characteristic, although if the femoral head overlies the acetabulum a subtle radiological sign may be that in a posterior dislocation, the femoral head

appears smaller than the normal, uninjured side, while in an anterior dislocation, the femoral head appears larger than the normal, uninjured side.

Management

An attempted closed reduction of the hip should be performed in the ER. In this situation as the patient is intubated and sedated, there is no need for conscious sedation. However, if the patient is awake, then conscious sedation is needed to adequately relax the patient in order to perform the reduction. There are multiple methods of reducing a hip for posterior dislocations; the Allis method is effective. The patient is placed supine on the table. The assistant holds down the pelvis and the surgeon stands on the table above the patient. The knee is flexed to 90+°, as well as the hip. The knee/lower leg is placed in between the surgeon's legs as upward traction is pulled; at the same time internal and external rotation of the hip is done. This will dislodge the hip from the posterior lip of the acetabulum and allow the joint to reduce. A 'clunk' is often felt and heard on successful reduction. The assistant can help by pushing on the femoral head, trying to coax it back into the acetabulum.

If closed reduction is unsuccessful, the patient should be taken to the operating theater for an attempt at closed reduction under general anesthesia where the patient will be more relaxed. If this is not successful then an open reduction is performed. For a posterior hip dislocation, the posterior Kocher-Langenbeck approach to the hip will provide adequate exposure and allow the sciatic nerve to be examined.

After successful reduction, the patient should be kept in an abduction brace or abduction pillow. The patient can start with partial weight bearing, and progress to weight bearing as tolerated while posterior dislocation precautions are maintained. Posterior precautions are avoiding any maneuver that will cause re-dislocation, such as internal rotation and adduction of the hip. This is often seen when patients bend over to tie their shoes.

Key points

- Posterior hip dislocations are more common than anterior hip dislocations and typically occur after high-energy trauma.
- They are often associated with fractures of the femoral head, neck and acetabulum, and sciatic nerve injuries. Commonly, the peroneal branch of the sciatic nerve is injured.
- Prior to reduction, a fracture of the femoral neck should be excluded.
- CT is sometimes obtained after closed reduction to assess for fractures and congruency of the hip joint.

References

1. Bucholz RW, Heckman JD, Court-Brown CM, *et al*, Eds. *Rockwood and Green's Fractures in Adults*, 6th ed. Philadelphia, PA: Lippincott Williams & Wilkins, 2006.

2. Brumback RJ, Kenzora JE, Levitt LE, Burgess AR, Poka A. Fractures of the femoral head. In: *The Hip Society*, ed. *Proceeding of the Hip Society*. St Louis, MO: Mosby, 1986: 181-206.

3. Thompson VP, Epstein HC. Traumatic dislocation of the hip; a survey of two hundred four cases covering a period of twenty-one years. *J Bone Joint Surg [Am]* 1951; 33: 746-78.

4. Pipkin G. Treatment of grade IV fracture-dislocation of the hip. *J Bone Joint Surg [Am]* 1957; 39: 1027-42.

Case 8

Clinical presentation

A 78-year-old woman sustains a mechanical fall at home after tripping on a step leading up to her kitchen. She falls on her right side, and is unable to subsequently ambulate. She is brought to the ER for further evaluation.

Physical examination

There is some bruising over the lateral right hip, with minimal swelling, and the skin is intact. The right leg is shortened and externally rotated compared with the left. There is tenderness to palpation in the groin. A femoral pulse is palpable. The patient has pain with attempted range of motion of the hip. When her knee is moved, she complains of pain in her hip. Distally, there are no neurovascular deficits.

Review the image below [Figure 19]. Describe your findings.

Questions

1. What is the diagnosis?

2. What is the mechanism of injury?

3. How are these injuries classified?

4. How is AVN staged?

5. Describe the blood supply of the femoral head. Why is this important?

6. Describe the anatomy of the three ligaments of the femoral neck.

7. What is Ward's triangle?

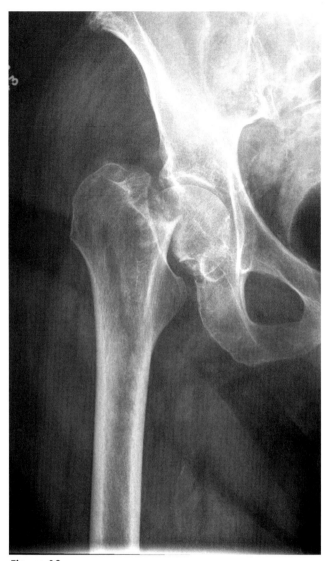

Figure 19.

Radiology findings

There is a complete subcapital fracture of the right proximal femur, with superior migration of the femoral shaft. The femoral head is detached from the femoral neck but remains within the acetabulum.

Answers

1. Garden grade IV subcapital femoral fracture.

2. In the elderly, the majority of femoral neck fractures are low-energy injuries occurring after a minor fall resulting in a direct blow to the greater trochanter or a fall with the extremity in external rotation. Younger patients are more likely to sustain a femoral neck fracture after high-energy trauma (for example, motor vehicle accidents). Cyclical loading-stress fractures of the femoral neck are also seen in population groups such as athletes, military recruits, and patients with osteoporosis.

3. Femoral neck fractures are classified according to the displacement of the proximal femoral head (the degree of valgus displacement), known as the Garden system. The system was devised based on the presence of distortion of the medial compressive trabeculae of the femoral head before reduction, as seen on AP radiographs:

   i) Garden I fractures are incomplete fractures with the femoral head in a valgus position;

   ii) Garden II fractures are complete fractures without displacement [Figure 20];

   iii) Garden III fractures are complete fractures with partial displacement of fracture fragments. The femoral head is in a varus position with medial rotation and there is external rotation of the femoral shaft;

   iv) Garden IV fractures are complete fractures with no contact between the fracture fragments [Figure 21]. There is shortening and external rotation of the femur, but the femoral head lies in its normal position within the acetabulum. The highest incidence of AVN is in groups III and IV.

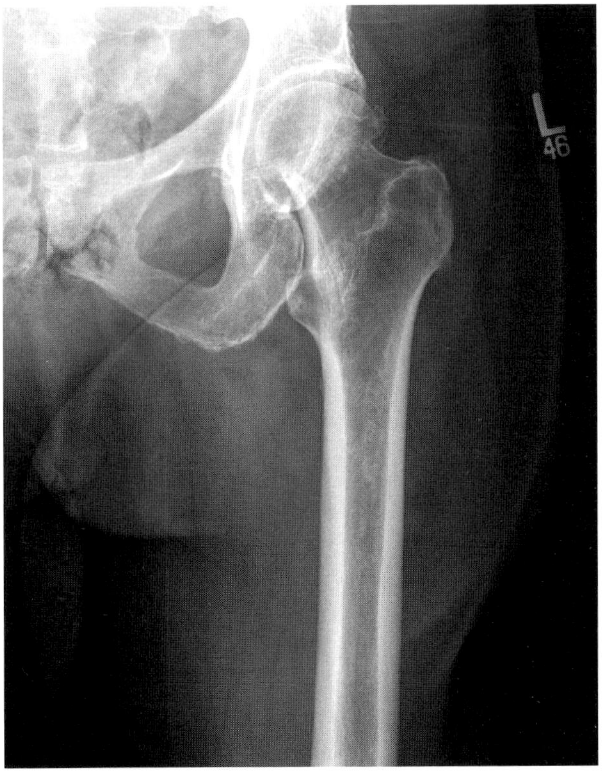

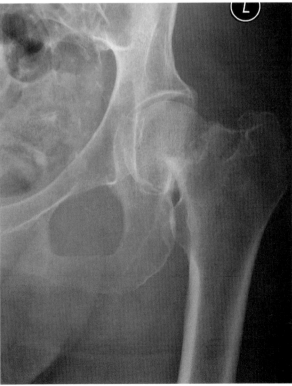

Figure 20. Garden II type fracture of the left femoral neck.

Figure 21. Garden IV type fracture of the left femoral neck.

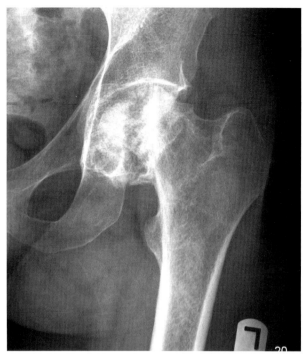

Figure 22. Ficat Stage 4 avascular necrosis of the left femoral head occurring as a complication of a subcapital fracture. There is sclerosis, joint space narrowing and collapse of the femoral head.

4. The Ficat and Arlet system is widely used to classify osteonecrosis (AVN) of the femoral head. It is based on plain film findings:

    i)   Stage 0 has no findings on plain films and is diagnosed by other imaging modalities such as a bone scan or MRI. It is also asymptomatic (making this a preclinical stage);

    ii) Stage 1 demonstrates patchy osteoporosis of the affected bone but without sclerosis. The patient complains of pain, and presents with restricted abduction and internal rotation at the hip joint;

    iii) Stage 2 manifests as patchy osteoporosis and sclerosis;

    iv) Stage 3 is progression of necrosis, with an abnormal contour of the femoral head and the presence of a crescent sign (curvilinear subchondral radiolucent line). This radiolucency is best appreciated at the anterolateral aspect of the proximal femoral head. There is preservation or a slight increase in the joint space;

    v)   Stage 4 is collapse of the femoral head, narrowing of the joint space and subchondral sclerosis [Figure 22]. On MR imaging, AVN is diagnosed when there is a band of low-signal intensity seen on all imaging sequences, best seen on T1-weighted images. On T2-weighted images, there may be high signal at the inner border of this peripheral band (called the 'double line' sign), which is pathognomonic for osteonecrosis [Figure 23].

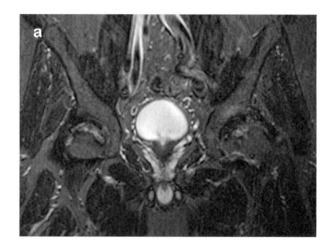

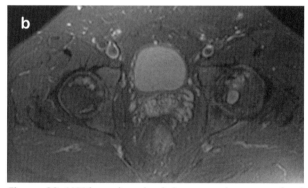

Figure 23. MRI imaging depicts avascular necrosis of the bilateral femoral heads.

5. The main blood supply to the femoral head comes from the profunda femoris artery, a branch of the femoral artery. Two branches, the medial femoral circumflex and the lateral femoral circumflex arteries, come from the profunda femoris artery and form an extracapsular ring

around the base of the femoral neck. The medial femoral circumflex artery curves posteriorly giving off some anterior cervical subcapsular branches, and the lateral femoral circumflex artery curves posteriorly giving off the majority of subcapsular arterial branches. This is important because a femoral neck fracture results in disruption of the blood supply to the femoral head. This can cause AVN of the head. The greater the displacement and the longer the time to reduction, the higher the risk of AVN. In young individuals, complete death of the femoral head is a challenge as the only effective treatments involve excision, arthrodesis or total hip replacement.

6. The three ligaments of the femoral neck are:
    i)   pubofemoral ligament: located anteriorly and connects the superior pubic ramus to the anterior-medial femoral neck;
    ii) Y-ligament of Bigelow (also known as the iliofemoral ligament): located anteriorly and connects the anterior inferior iliac spine to the intertrochanteric region of the femoral neck;
    iii) ischiofemoral ligament: located posteriorly and connects the body of the ischium to the posterior femoral neck.
    The anatomy of the capsular ligaments is important, because, as noted above, the capsular ligaments connect the femoral head and neck to the pelvis, but not really to the femoral shaft. Most of the distal attachment of the femoral head and neck is anterior; there is little ligamentous stability posteriorly. The ligament that is the strongest is the Y-ligament of Bigelow, and it also has the most distal attachment. Therefore, for there to be significant displacement of the femoral neck, this ligament is usually injured.

7. Ward's triangle is an area on plain film that is devoid of trabeculae. It is located in the middle of the femoral neck, just above the intertrochanteric line. The trabeculae form in a manner that reflects the stresses applied across the bone. The lateral femoral neck sustains the tension forces applied across the femur as there is progressive weight bearing. Vertically oriented trabeculae are seen here, indicative of tensile stress. The compressive side of the femoral neck is the medial side. This is also where the abductor muscles apply their force. Horizontal trabeculae are seen on the compressive side, indicative of adduction and compression. The vertical and horizontal trabeculae cross at right angles, except for at Ward's triangle where they do not cross at all, hence, the apparent lack of trabeculae on X-ray. The Garden system of classifying femoral neck fractures is based on the alignment of these trabeculae. When there is a femoral neck fracture, the horizontal trabeculae will show a beak or angle at the fracture line. In Garden I fractures, the horizontal trabeculae of the femoral head and neck are slightly angled into valgus at the fracture line. In Garden II fractures, the fracture is non-displaced, and the trabeculae remain aligned. In Garden III fractures, there is fixed angulation between the fracture fragments so there is a marked varus angulation at the fracture line, and the trabeculae in the head fragment are angled out of the normal position. In Garden IV fractures, there is no contact between the fracture fragments and the trabeculae of the head lie in their normal anatomical position but there is no connection with the head and neck fragment.

Management

These fractures are treated surgically in order to allow early return to function, decrease the risk of femoral head osteonecrosis in younger patients and to allow early mobility of the patient in the elderly.

In young individuals, the goal is to save the femoral head to avoid the need for a hip replacement early in life. This is done by early surgery, reducing the fracture, and placing three parallel screws from the femoral neck into the head, but not penetrating the joint. The reduction is usually achieved on the traction table by traction and internal rotation, while some surgeons prefer to flex the hip, and apply axial traction and external rotation. This will unlock the fracture fragment while subsequent internal rotation and hip extension should reduce the fragment. Once adequate reduction is achieved, the three screws are inserted, although some surgeons rely on two screws only. Traditionally the most stable construct is that of an inverted triangle, with one screw near the inferior femoral neck, and one near the posterior femoral neck. Screws should be placed above the lesser trochanter to avoid the risk of creating a subtrochanteric stress riser. In young patients many surgeons prefer an open reduction.

In elderly individuals with poor bone quality, screw fixation is not useful and replacement of the femoral head with a hemiarthroplasty is performed. If the patient is very active or younger, a total hip replacement should be considered.

Key points

- Intracapsular fractures include fractures of the femoral neck and head with capital, subcapital, transcervical, and basicervical types.

- The Garden system is used to classify fractures of the femoral neck. This is based on the amount of displacement of the femoral neck, which can be identified by following the alignment of the trabeculae.

- These fractures are treated by percutaneous screw fixation, hemiarthroplasty or total hip arthroplasty depending on the patient's biological age, lifestyle, and bone quality.

References

1. Ficat RP. Idiopathic bone necrosis of the femoral head: early diagnosis and treatment. *J Bone Joint Surg [Br]* 1985; 67: 3-9.

2. Mitchell DG, Rao VM, Dalinka MK, *et al.* Femoral head avascular necrosis: correlation of MR imaging, radiographic staging, radionuclide imaging and clinical findings. *Radiology* 1987; 162: 709-15.

3. Pappas JN. The musculoskeletal crescent sign. *Radiology* 2000; 217(1): 213-4.

4. Kyle RF. Fractures of the hip. In: *Fractures and Dislocations*, Vol 2. Gustilo RB, Kyle RF, Templeman DC, Eds. St. Louis, MO: Mosby-Yearbook, 1993: 770-831.

Case 9

Clinical presentation

An 82-year-old woman presents to the ER after she tripped and fell over her rug in the middle of the night when waking up to get a glass of water. She noted immediate pain in her left hip after the fall, and subsequently was unable to get up or bear weight. She presents to the ER complaining of pain in her left groin.

Physical examination

On exam, the skin around her left hip is intact. There is mild swelling, and no bruising. Her left lower extremity is shortened and externally rotated. She has pain with range of motion of her hip. Distally, there are no neurovascular deficits.

Review the image below [Figure 24]. Describe your findings.

Questions

1. What is the likely diagnosis?

2. What is the mechanism of injury?

3. How are these injuries classified?

4. Why are isolated lesser trochanteric fractures important?

5. What complications may occur?

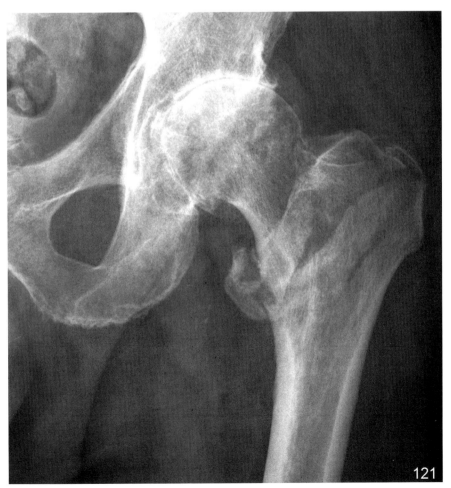

Figure 24.

Radiology findings

There is a comminuted intertrochanteric fracture as well as avulsion of the lesser trochanter with severe osteoarthritis of the hip.

Answers

1. Intertrochanteric fracture.

2. In young patients, intertrochanteric fractures are seen in high-energy injuries, such as motor vehicle accidents. In the elderly, these fractures are seen in low-energy injuries, such as a simple fall. These patients are slow ambulators, and therefore tend to fall on their sides instead of face forward like young children learning how to walk. As the elderly individual falls on his/her side, they land on the greater trochanter. The area has decreased fat and muscle mass, absorbs the force, and transmits it to bone of poor quality, which then fractures. These individuals are often osteoporotic and there may be other associated injuries, such as a fracture of the distal humerus or proximal humerus.

3. The commonly used classification system for intertrochanteric fractures is the Evans system, which is based on the stability of the fracture pattern [Figure 25]. The system is centered around the idea that a stable reduction of an intertrochanteric fracture is dependent on restoration of the posteromedial femoral cortex. Stable and unstable fracture patterns are divided into two groups. In stable patterns, the posteromedial cortex remains intact or is only minimally comminuted. In unstable patterns, there is greater comminution of the posteromedial cortex. These injuries can be converted into stable ones if medial cortical apposition is achieved during reduction.

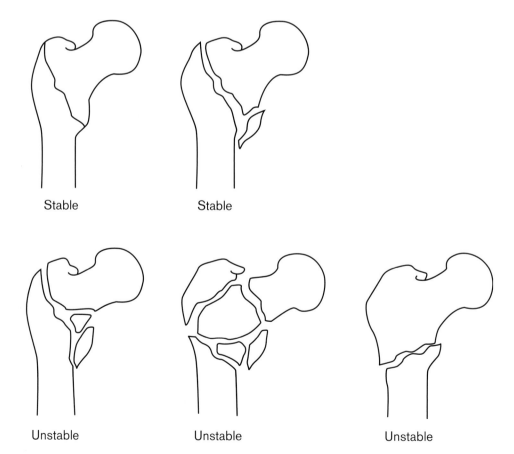

Stable   Stable

Unstable   Unstable   Unstable

Figure 25. Evans classification of intertrochanteric fractures.

4. In adolescents, isolated lesser trochanteric fractures are common avulsion-type injuries, and occur due to forceful iliopsoas contracture. In the elderly, however, isolated lesser trochanter fractures are pathologic lesions of the proximal femur until proven otherwise [Figures 26 and 27].

5. A variety of complications may occur including non-union, loss of fixation, AVN, neurovascular injury (for example, laceration of the superficial femoral artery due to a displaced lesser trochanter fragment) and post-traumatic osteoarthritis.

Management

These injuries are functionally debilitating, and are corrected surgically. Ideally, patients are treated within the first 48-72 hours of injury, as studies have shown increased mortality in the elderly when fixation is delayed beyond this time. The goal of treatment is to allow the patient early return to function without technical failure of the implant. This depends on the bone quality, nature of the fracture, choice of implant, and the quality of the reduction. Multiple surgical fixation options are available depending on the nature of the fracture. Unstable fractures are usually seen in elderly women who are dependent ambulators/dependent on others for care. These patients are of increased age, and due to their already poor functional status combined with age, are likely to have poor quality bone lending them to this type of fracture after a fall. An unstable fracture is also one which involves the posteromedial cortex, as described above.

A stable fracture can be treated with a compression hip screw. Unstable fractures can be treated by multiple means, such as a trochanteric stabilizing plate, an axial compression hip screw, or an intramedullary hip screw.

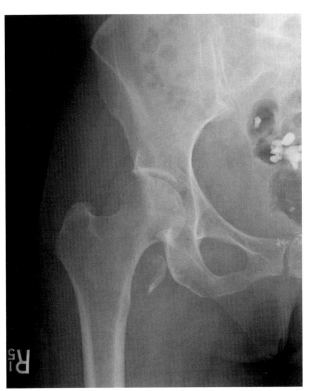

Figure 26. Avulsion fracture of the right lesser trochanter in a 56-year-old female.

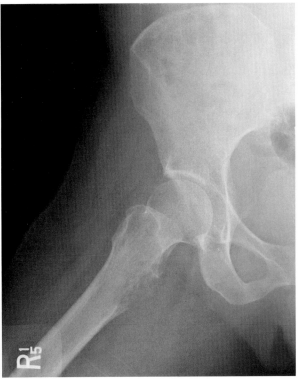

Figure 27. There is a permeative pattern of bone destruction at the region of the lesser trochanter extended into the medullary cavity. There is a wide zone of transition giving it an aggressive appearance. The patient was found to have metastatic disease from primary lung cancer.

Stable fracture

◆ Compression hip screw. To reduce the fracture axial traction is applied, which restores length and unlocks fracture fragments. Varus deformity is corrected. A neck shaft angle between 5° varus and 20° of valgus is considered acceptable. Very little angulation is acceptable on a lateral view. To ensure correct rotation of the femur, the amount of femoral anteversion on lateral X-ray is compared with the patella. 15-20° of anteversion of the femur is within normal limits.

Unstable fracture

◆ Compression hip screw. This is widely used and generally successful, accepting that there may be significant collapse and excessive medialization in the most unstable cases. This normally facilitates healing but may produce troublesome local muscle imbalance, gross shortening and poor bone healing. This is not indicated for reverse obliquity or subtrochanteric fractures.

◆ Compression hip screw with additional trochanteric stabilization plate. The trochanteric stabilization plate is added to the lateral side of the compression hip screw to restrict excessive slide and medialization.

◆ Combination sliding plate - the Medoff plate. This allows controlled shortening of the femoral neck and upper shaft to facilitate healing. It is successful in some surgeons' hands but not widely used.

◆ 95° fixed angle blade/screw. These devices are not used for primary trochanteric fractures as it will not allow slide and is more invasive. They are useful for primary plating of a reverse obliquity fracture, subtrochanteric fracture, or non-union.

◆ Intramedullary 'sliding screw' fixation. Many nails are now available, the gamma nail, trochanteric fixation nail (TFN), or the intramedullary hip screw (IMHS) being common examples. These are becoming much more popular and are very successful. They allow controlled collapse until the fracture rests on the proximal end of the nail which maintains some proximal femoral anatomy.

After surgery, patients are made to weight bear as tolerated to allow early return of function. Most patients will require some form of physical therapy and extensive rehabilitation in order to return to pre-injury function.

Key points

◆ Extracapsular fractures include intertrochanteric and subtrochanteric fractures.

◆ Intertrochanteric fractures are divided into stable and unstable injuries. Unstable fractures are those with disruption of the posteromedial cortex, and fractures in patients likely to have poor bone quality.

◆ Unlike intracapsular fractures of the hip, AVN is a rare complication because they occur in cancellous bone with extensive blood supply.

◆ Basicervical fractures are just proximal or at the intertrochanteric line. They are extracapsular and carry a greater risk of AVN.

References

1. Evans E. The treatment of trochanteric fractures of the femur. *J Bone Joint Surg* 1949; 31B: 190-203.

2. Bertin KC, Horstman J, Coleman SS. Isolated fracture of the lesser trochanter in adults: an initial manifestation of metastatic malignant disease. *J Bone Joint Surg* 1984; 66A: 770-3.

3. Gradwohl JR, Mailliard JA. Cough-induced avulsion of the lesser trochanter. *Neb Med J* 1987; August: 280-1.

4. Phillips C, Pope T, Jones J, *et al.* Nontraumatic avulsion of the lesser trochanter: a pathognomonic sign of metastatic disease. *Skeletal Radiol* 1988; 17: 106-10.

5. Baumgaertner L. Unstable intertrochanteric hip fractures in the elderly. *J Am Acad Orthop Surg* 2004; 12: 179-90.

Case 10

Clinical presentation

A 42-year-old man presents to the ER after a high-speed motor vehicle collision. He was alert and oriented at the scene, and hemodynamically stable at the scene. His presentation is similar in the trauma bay, except now the patient is slightly tachycardic. His left thigh is swollen and tender. The orthopaedic team are aware of a high-speed trauma coming to the hospital, and are present as part of the trauma team to aid in the trauma evaluation.

Physical examination

On physical exam the patient's left leg is swollen anteriorly over the thigh. The skin is intact, but has multiple superficial lacerations. The patient will not allow you to move his hip or knee. Proximally, he has a palpable femoral artery pulse, and distally you are able to palpate a dorsalis pedis and posterior tibial artery pulse. He is able to dorsiflex and plantar flex his ankle, and he can extend his great toe. His vital signs are stable and he is otherwise uninjured.

Review the images below [Figures 28 and 29]. Describe your findings.

Questions

1. What is the diagnosis?

2. What is the mechanism of injury?

3. What are some associated injuries?

4. Why may this patient be tachycardic in the trauma bay?

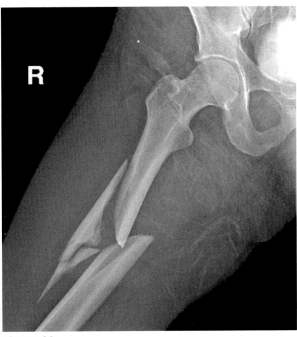

Figure 28.

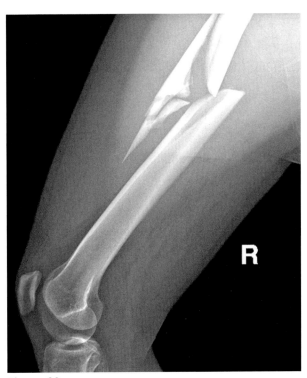

Figure 29.

Radiology fndings

There is a comminuted midshaft femur fracture, with a butterfly fragment.

Answers

1. Femoral shaft fracture.

2. Fractures of the femoral shaft are seen in both younger and older patients. In younger patients, the mechanism is usually high-energy trauma such as a motor vehicle crash. In older patients (especially elderly, osteoporotic women), the mechanism is more often a simple, low-energy fall. In young athletes, stress fractures of the femoral shaft should be considered.

3. Femur fractures are high-energy injuries, therefore, distant and local associated traumatic injuries should also be searched for, such as pelvic injuries and spinal injuries. In particular with the femur, it is important to exclude an ipsilateral acetabular fracture, a femoral neck fracture, and/or a distal femur fracture. Combination injuries involving the neck and shaft are particularly easy to miss (the femoral neck element) on initial X-rays but can significantly complicate treatment.

4. Femur fractures alone can lead to significant blood loss into the thigh which is capable of holding several units of blood. This patient may be tachycardic due to blood loss in his thigh, but given the mechanism of injury other areas of potential bleeding should also be evaluated.

Management

The treatment of choice for a femoral shaft fracture is operative with insertion of a reamed femoral nail.

Initial application of traction will help alleviate pain, muscle spasm and temporarily maintain length. A tamponade effect will help reduce blood loss.

Definitive fixation is usually done using an intrameduallary nail. This can be inserted antegrade or retrograde. Antegrade insertion is performed via the piriformis fossa or occasionally via the greater trochanter as the starting point. The femur is bowed anteriorly, and this bowing is taken into account when the nail is inserted. Retrograde nailing is inserted through an intercondylar entry point. The nails are locked distally and proximally to control shaft rotation. The union rate is in the order of 95%.

Key points

♦   **A fracture of the femoral shaft is one which occurs 5cm distal to the lesser trochanter and 5cm proximal to the adductor tubercle.**

♦   **The gold standard of treatment is antegrade femoral nailing inserted through a reamed technique.**

♦   **These injuries may initially be placed in femoral traction to maintain position and provide initial comfort.**

References

1.   Koval KJ, Zuckerman JD. Femoral shaft. In: *Handbook of Fractures*, 2nd ed. Philadelphia, PA: Lippincott, Williams and Wilkins, 2002: 212-7.

2.   Thompson JC. Thigh/hip. In: *Netter's Concise Atlas of Orthopedic Anatomy*. Icon Learning Systems Inc., 2002: 167-98.

3.   Ertl JP, Ertl WJ. Femur injuries and fractures. eMedicine. Available at: http://www.emedicine.com/sports/topic38.htm. Accessed October 31, 2008.

Case 11

Clinical presentation

A 76-year-old female presents after having been recently discharged from the hospital after undergoing a left total hip replacement ten days ago. She woke up in the middle of the night to go to the bathroom, tripped over the rug and fell. Immediately afterwards she noticed pain in her left thigh and knee, and was unable to bear weight. She did not hit her head, and she did not lose consciousness. The patient only has one injury, as shown below.

Physical examination

Her left thigh is swollen, but soft. She has pain with range of motion. Distally, her knee appears benign, without an effusion, tenderness, or gross deformity. When a range of motion for the knee is attempted, she splints, complaining of pain in her left thigh. She reports no groin pain. The skin is intact. Distally, she has a palpable posterial tibial and dorsalis pedis pulse, and is SILT (sensation intact to light touch) L4/L5/S1.

Review the image below [Figure 30]. Describe your findings.

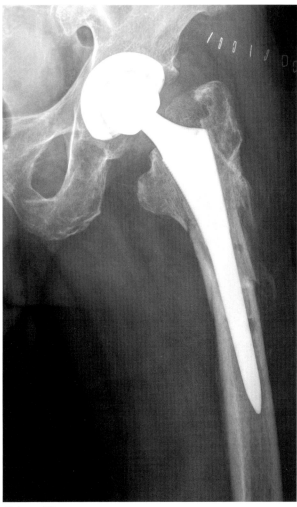

Figure 30.

Questions

1. What is the diagnosis?

2. What is the mechanism of injury?

3. What is the Vancouver classification system?

4. Based on this patient's history, physical exam, and X-rays, what are her risk factors for having this injury, and how would this help you classify it?

Radiology findings

There is a comminuted fracture of the proximal femur surrounding the total hip prosthesis, which was not present on the postoperative film ten days prior [Figure 31]. It involves the lesser trochanter as well as the proximal shaft around the stem of the prosthesis. The acetabular component is satisfactory. There is no evidence of dislocation.

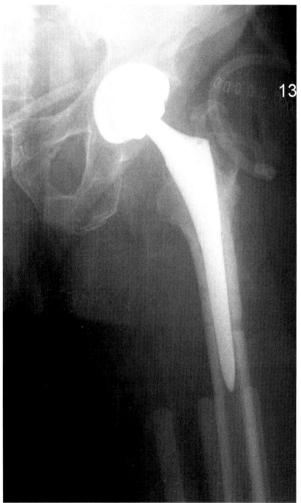

Figure 31. Initial postoperative film taken ten days prior demonstrates an intact proximal femur.

Answers

1. Periprosthetic fracture about a total hip replacement.

2. Periprosthetic hip fractures generally occur after minor trauma, such as a low-energy mechanical fall, as seen in this patient. Revision surgery has also been sited as a cause for periprosthetic fractures.

3. There are multiple methods to describe periprosthetic fractures. The Vancouver classification system is one of the most commonly used. The system functions by describing where the fracture is in relation to the prosthesis, and the quality of bone involved:
   i) Type A: fractures around the trochanter:
      ◆ A-L involves the lesser trochanter (more likely to lead to instability);
      ◆ A-G involves the greater trochanter (stable, higher association with osteolysis);
   ii) Type B: fractures around the femoral stem:
      ◆ B1 fractures - stable implant, good quality bone;
      ◆ B2 fractures - loose implant, good quality bone;
      ◆ B3 fractures - loose implant, poor quality bone;
   iii) Type C: fractures distal to the femoral stem.

4. Risk factors for this patient are that she is osteopenic (as is expected from her age, and noted on her X-rays), and underwent recent surgery. Because she fell and broke through after recently having the implant placed, the most likely explanation is that the implant was loose. The combination of poor bone quality with a loose implant can explain why she has a periprosthetic fracture after a low-energy fall. This is a Vancouver Type B fracture, specifically a B3.

Management

Periprosthetic fractures are complicated, and require specialist management. The Vancouver classification helps guide treatment:

◆ Type A. With a fracture of the greater trochanter, there may be decreased abductor function. A wire can be placed around the trochanter for fixation. A fracture of the lesser trochanter can be associated with implant loosening, and may require revision.

- Type B. If the implant is stable, revision is not needed. The fracture can be fixed using the appropriate method of fixation for the fracture type. The presence of the implant in the canal modifies the treatment requirement. If the implant is loose, but the bone is good quality, a revision to a longer stemmed implant may be adequate. If the implant is loose and the bone is of poor quality, then a more complex revision with an appropriate method of fixation may be required.
- Type C. Here the fracture is well away from the implant. Therefore, the implant can be left alone, and the fracture can be fixed appropriately.

Key points

- Loose implants account for approximately one third of periprosthetic fractures.
- In revision surgery, the new implant should be located distally two shaft widths below the old implant in order to get stable fixation.
- Risk factors for periprosthetic fractures include osteopenia, revision surgery, stress risers, and improper femoral stem preparation.

References

1. Duncan CP, Masri BA. Fractures of the femur after hip replacement. In: *Instructional Course Lectures 44*. Jackson D, Ed. Rosemont, IL: American Academy of Orthopaedic Surgeons, 1995: 293-304.

2. Koval KJ, Zukerman JD. *Handbook of Fractures*, 3rd ed. Philadelphia, PA: Lippincott Williams & Wilkins, 2006: 41-4

3. Bucholz RW, Heckman JD, Court-Brown CM, *et al*. Eds. *Rockwood and Green's Fractures in Adults*, 6th ed. Philadelphia, PA: Lippincott Williams & Wilkins, 2006.

Case 12

Clinical presentation

A 76-year-old woman presents after sustaining a fall at home after slipping in her kitchen and landing on her left knee. She notes pain and swelling at her left knee, and is unable to ambulate. She is brought to the ER by her daughter for further evaluation. On discussion with the daughter, it is discovered that her mother has fallen previously on her left leg, sustaining a femoral fracture which required an orthopedic procedure.

Physical examination

On exam, there is diffuse swelling at the distal femur extending over the knee. There is ecchymosis, but the skin is intact. Her left leg appears slightly shorter than her right leg. A scar is noted proximally from a previous procedure on the lateral aspect of the femur. There is no pain with range of motion of the hip, but the patient complains of knee pain when her femur is moved. Distally, she will not allow anyone to move her knee. There is tenderness over the distal femur. There are no neurovascular deficits.

Review the image below [Figure 32]. Describe your findings.

Questions

1. What is the diagnosis?

2. What is the mechanism of injury?

3. Describe the anatomy of the distal femur.

4. What muscle groups are acting to displace this fracture?

5. What is the AO classification for this fracture?

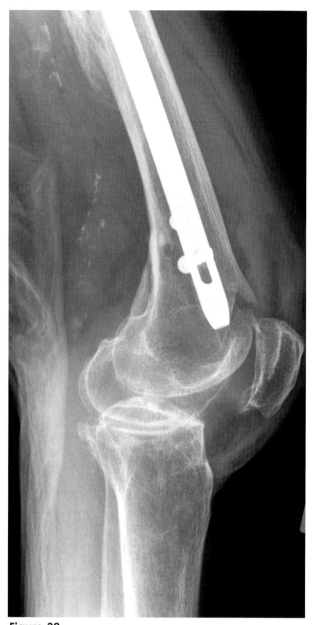

Figure 32.

Radiology findings

There is an oblique comminuted supracondylar fracture of the distal femoral metaphysis, traversing the location of the distal fixation screw of the intramedullary nail. A joint effusion is evident, as well as severe degenerative changes. A CT sagittal image demonstrates the oblique path of the fracture line from posterosuperior to anteroinferior at the level of the superior margin of the patella [Figure 33]. Axial imaging further confirms the degree of comminution [Figure 34]. Of note, this new fracture is distinct from the previous femoral midshaft fracture, now demonstrating interval callus formation.

Answers

1. Periprosthetic distal femur fracture about the distal locking screws of a femoral intramedullary nail.

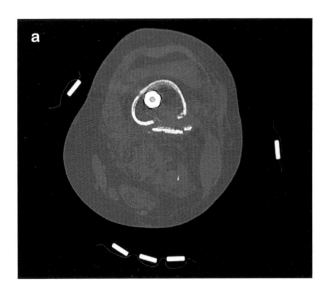

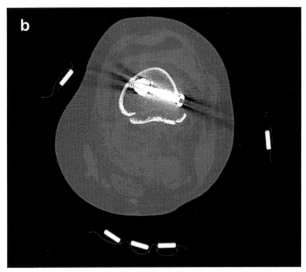

Figure 34. Axial CT images demonstrate a comminuted fracture of the distal femoral metaphysis centered on an intramedullary femoral nail.

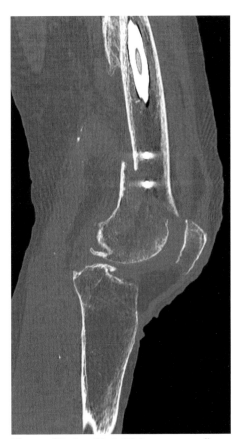

Figure 33. Sagittal CT image confirms an oblique fracture of the distal femoral metaphysis.

2. In the elderly, supracondylar femoral fractures are usually low energy, resulting from a fall onto a flexed knee. Axial load is transmitted through poor quality bone, causing a fracture. In young adults, this injury is due to high-energy trauma, such as a motor vehicle accident.

3. The distal femur is divided into supracondylar and condylar regions. This fracture is an oblique fracture, lying in the supracondylar region. The distal femur is trapezoidal in shape. This is because the condyles are wider posteriorly than

anteriorly. The anatomic axis of the femur is valgus angulated by 7-11°; this is caused by the medial condyle being more convex and extending more distal compared with the lateral condyle. On the lateral view, the lateral femoral cortex is aligned with the lateral condyle. In the axial view, the lateral condyle is inclined approximately 10° and the medial condyle approximately 25°.

4. While several muscles cross the knee the primary displacing force is the unopposed flexion of the distal fragment by the gastrocnemius which originates from the posterior surfaces of the femoral condyles.

5. In the AO classification, articular fractures are classified as either:
    i)   Type A: non-articular (i.e., involving only the supracondylar portion);
    ii) Type B: partial articular (a shearing fracture extending through only part of the joint); or
    iii) Type C: a complete articular fracture with a fracture passing into the joint and a fracture separating the whole of the joint from the rest of the bone. In this case, the fracture does not appear to involve the articular surface, and therefore can be classified as an A type fracture.

Management

There are many ways to manage distal femur fractures. With this fracture, the additional hardware causes difficulties. The involved hardware is likely to be an intramedullary nail for a femoral shaft fracture. If this fracture is mature and healed, it may be possible to remove the nail and routinely reconstruct the distal femur. If the nail has to be maintained in position, a device can be chosen that may be able to bypass the nail. A 'LISS' plate (less invasive stabilization system [Synthes]) can be used for this type of fracture. The position or length of some of the screws of the new implant may need to be modified to accommodate the pre-existing nail.

After surgery range of motion of the joint is allowed as tolerated. However, weight bearing is restricted. The patient is kept touch-down weight bearing for approximately 8-12 weeks, or until there is adequate radiographic evidence of healing. To help with postoperative stability, the knee is often placed in a hinged knee brace.

Key points

♦   **The distal femur is not symmetric laterally, medially, or anteriorly and posteriorly. It is wider posteriorly than anteriorly, angled more medially than laterally, and the medial condyle is longer than the lateral condyle.**

♦   **Distal femur fractures are usually low-energy injuries in the elderly, and high-energy injuries in the young.**

♦   **Periprosthetic fractures can be stabilized adequately with modern devices but the surgery may need to be individualized based on the fracture anatomy and the presence of previous implants.**

♦   **Postoperative weight bearing is guarded, but the joint should be stable enough after fixation to encourage a free range of motion.**

References

1. Culp RW, Schmidt RG, Hanks G, et al. Supracondylar fracture of the femur following prosthetic knee arthroplasty. Clin Orthop 1987; (222): 212-22.

2. Figgie MP, Goldberg VM, Figgie HE 3rd, et al. The results of treatment of supracondylar fracture above total knee arthroplasty. J Arthroplasty 1990; 5(3): 267-76.

3. Schmotzer H, Tchejeyan GH, Dall DM. Surgical management of intra- and postoperative fractures of the femur about the tip of the stem in total hip arthroplasty. J Arthroplasty 1996; 11(6): 709-17.

4. Sisto DJ, Lachiewicz PF, Insall JN. Treatment of supracondylar fractures following prosthetic arthroplasty of the knee. Clin Orthop 1985; (196): 265-72.

5. Lindahl H, Garellick G, Regner H, Herberts P, Malchau H. Three hundred and twenty-one periprosthetic femoral fractures. J Bone Joint Surg [Am] 2006; 88: 1215-22.

6. Lindahl H, Malchau H, Oden A, Garellick G. Risk factors for failure after treatment of a periprosthetic fracture of the femur. J Bone Joint Surg [Br] 2006; 88-B: 26-30.

7. Klein GR, Parvizi J, Rapuri V, Wolf CF, Hozack WJ, Sharkey PF, Purtill JJ. Proximal femoral replacement for the treatment of periprosthetic fractures. J Bone Joint Surg [Am] 2005; 87: 1777-81.

Chapter 7

Knee and leg

Case 1

Clinical presentation

An otherwise healthy 56-year-old man presents with an injury to his knee. While jumping down a few steps, he felt/heard a 'snap' in his leg, and immediately fell to the ground. He was able to stand up afterwards, but noted that his knee was swollen, and that it was too painful to bear weight. There are no other complaints.

Physical examination

His knee is diffusely swollen and tender to palpation. There appears to be a gap in the patella. He is unable to actively extend his knee or straight leg raise. It is unclear if this is due to pain or due to damage to his extensor mechanism. He has a palpable popliteal pulse, and normal distal circulation. There are no neurologic deficits.

Review the images below [Figures 1 and 2]. Describe your findings.

Questions

1. What is the diagnosis?

2. How are these injuries classified?

3. Describe the various mechanisms of injury that can result in this fracture.

4. What types of complications can occur from these injuries?

5. What other injuries should you look for?

6. What normal patellar configuration should be distinguished from this injury?

7. Briefly describe the anatomy around the knee.

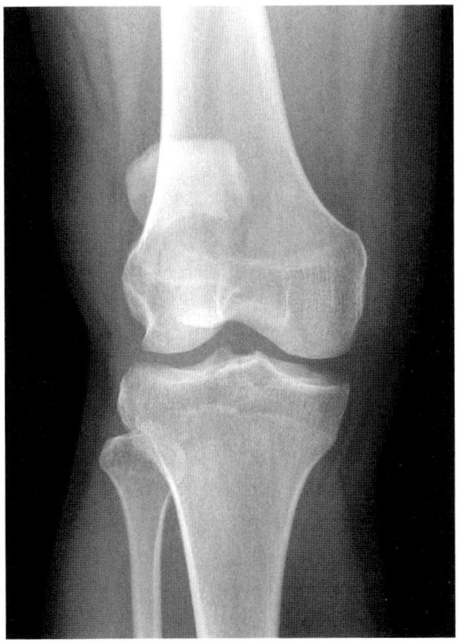

![Figure 1 radiograph]

Figure 1.

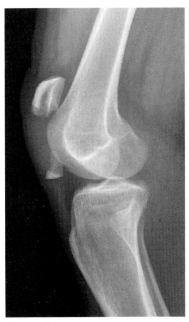

Figure 2.

Radiology findings

Plain film radiographs of the knee show a transverse fracture through the inferior portion of the patella with marked distraction of fracture fragments. There is superior displacement of the superior pole (by the quadriceps tendon) and inferior displacement of the inferior pole (by the patellar tendon). There is no evidence of an effusion or lipohemarthrosis, as the whole joint capsule is disrupted.

Answers

1. Transverse patellar fracture.

2. A basic classification system includes whether the fracture is open or closed, and non-displaced or displaced. Displaced fractures are defined as a minimum of 3mm of separation of fracture fragments or a minimum of 2mm of

articular incongruity. Patellar fractures are also further classified by descriptive terms. Transverse fractures are most common, dividing the patella into a superior and inferior fragment and usually involve the central or distal third of the patella [Figure 3]. Vertical fractures are less common, and occur in the superior to inferior direction. A stellate or multifragmented pattern is common. Fractures may also involve the inferior or superior poles. Osteochondral fractures are avulsion injuries of any part of the patellar articular surface (usually the inferior pole) and may be associated with patellar dislocation or subluxation.

3. Patellar fractures can result secondary to direct or indirect trauma. A direct blow is typically seen after a fall onto the knee or in a motor vehicle accident, with the patella hitting the dashboard. Indirect trauma to the patella occurs after a jump or after rapid unexpected knee flexion. Often, patellar fractures result from a combined indirect/direct mechanism.

4. Non-union, malunion and delayed union are potential complications of patellar fractures. Avascular necrosis may occur, as well as post-traumatic arthritis and/or quadriceps tendon weakness. Other potential complications include chondromalacia, arthrofibrosis of the knee joint, and infection.

5. Associated injuries should be suspected according to the mechanism of injury. Direct blows (dashboard injuries) may be associated with femoral shaft and neck fractures and hip dislocation. Indirect mechanism injuries are usually isolated but a more complex knee injury may be present. These include injuries involving the cruciate ligaments, tibial plateau or menisci. An occult knee dislocation should be considered.

6. A bipartite patella should be distinguished from a true patellar fracture [Figure 4]. It looks like an old non-displaced fracture, commonly in the superolateral corner of the patella. It is frequently bilateral and has smooth, rounded margins.

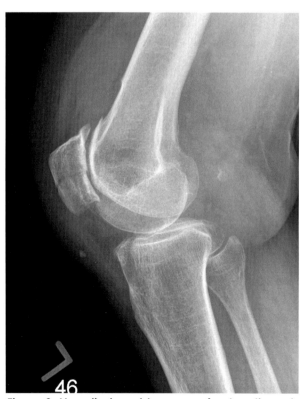

Figure 3. Non-displaced transverse fracture through the central portion of the patella.

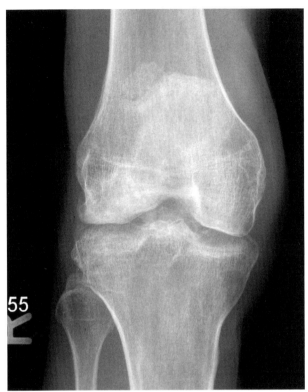

Figure 4. Typical appearance of a bipartite patella, occurring in the superolateral corner.

7. Anatomy around the patella is as follows:
    i)   superior pole = site of attachment of trilaminar quadriceps tendon (superficial rectus femoris, vastus intermedius, vastus medialis and vastus lateralis);
    ii) inferior pole = site of attachment of patellar tendon that then attaches to the anterior lip of the tibial tubercle;
    iii) medially = medial retinaculum (vastus medialis, rectus femoris);
    iv) laterally = lateral retinaculum (vastus lateralis).

Management

Fracture management is based on the integrity of the extensor mechanism. If the patient can straight leg raise, non-operative management is indicated. If not, surgical reconstruction is required. Patellar fractures can be treated non-operatively if the fracture is minimally displaced (<2mm) and the extensor mechanism is found to be intact. Non-operative treatment involves bracing in extension, crutches, no heavy physical activity, and weight bearing as tolerated. Acutely, it is difficult to evaluate the extensor mechanism in the emergent setting due to pain. The patient can be treated conservatively with pain medication, a knee immobilizer, and crutches. Upon a return visit when swelling and inflammation have decreased, a more thorough exam of the extensor mechanism can be undertaken.

Operative reconstruction does not need to be done emergently. The patient can be given a knee immobilizer and crutches in the ER, and told to follow-up within a week with his orthopedist to arrange surgical fixation. Reconstruction normally involves tension band wire fixation sometimes through a cannulated screw. Fracture fragments not amenable to fixation may be removed in the operating theater.

Key points

◆ Patellar fractures are typically transverse in orientation and are caused by direct or indirect trauma.

◆ Loss of extensor mechanism function is the key issue; displacement of 2mm or more is less important.

References

1. Bucholz RW, Heckman JD, Court-Brown CM, *et al*, Eds. *Rockwood and Green's Fractures in Adults*, 6th ed. Philadelphia, PA: Lippincott Williams & Wilkins, 2006.

2. Christine Lamoureaux, 'patella, fractures' Department of Radiology, Rocky Mountain medical imaging. www.emedicine .com.

Case 2

Clinical presentation

A 23-year-old male presents to the ER after jumping out of a third floor window. His room mates, who witnessed the fall, report that their friend landed on his feet and then fell to the ground immediately afterwards. At the scene he is conversant, but confused. In the trauma bay he continues to be confused, and is found to be tachycardic. His right knee is swollen and deformed. He has no other obvious injuries.

Physical examination

On exam, the right knee is grossly swollen and deformed compared with the left knee. The local skin is intact. Distally, there are no dorsalis pedis or posterior tibial pulses. Posterior to the knee, there is too much swelling and deformity to find a popliteal pulse. The patient, although confused, is in severe pain and is unwilling to move his ankle or toes.

Review the images below [Figures 5 and 6]. Describe your findings.

Questions

1. What is the diagnosis?

2. How do these injuries occur?

3. What other injures might be present?

4. How are these injuries classified?

5. What tests can you perform to assess ligamentous stability?

6. When may low-energy knee dislocations occur?

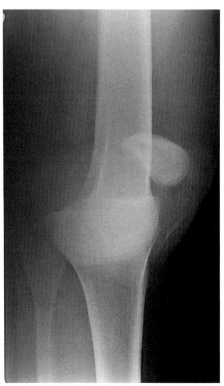

Figure 5.

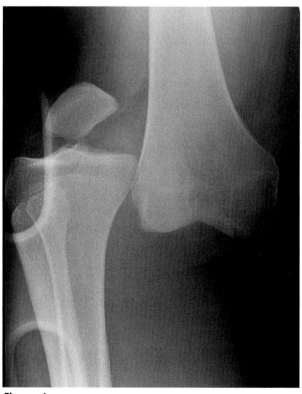

Figure 6.

Radiology findings

There is complete dislocation of the knee. No acute fractures are noted.

Answers

1. Knee dislocation.

2. Knee dislocations occur mainly in two directions. An anterior dislocation is due to a hyperextension injury, and is more common than posterior knee dislocations. Posterior knee dislocations occur due to axial loading on a flexed knee, such as a knee striking a dashboard during a high-speed motor vehicle collision.

3. In a complete knee dislocation, there is associated disruption of all of the four main ligaments of the knee. In partial injuries, most commonly the anterior (ACL) and posterior cruciate ligaments (PCL) are torn. The main risk is damage to the vasculature with disruption of the popliteal artery. Any difference in distal pulse pressure suggests a critical arterial injury and should be acutely investigated and managed. Compartment syndrome is also important to watch out for. There may also be other concomitant fractures involving the femur, acetabulum, and tibial plateau. Finally, neurological injury may occur, most commonly involving the peroneal nerve.

4. Knee dislocations are commonly classified according to a descriptive system, which describes the dislocation based on displacement of the proximal tibia relative to the distal femur (devised by Kennedy in 1963). In this system, there are five types of knee dislocations: anterior, posterior, lateral, medial and rotational. The mechanism of injury partly determines the type of dislocation that will most likely occur. For example, a hyperextension injury results in anterior dislocation whereas a flexion injury results in posterior dislocation. Anterior dislocations are most common and are associated with PCL injuries, and occasional ACL injuries.

5. There are various tests to examine for injured knee ligaments; many will be impossible in this scenario due to pain and marked frank instability:

i) ACL: injured if the patient has a positive Lachman's test in slight flexion of the knee. The Lachman's test is performed by placing one hand on the back of the femur, and the other on top of the distal tibia. The tibia and femur are displaced anteriorly and posteriorly in opposite directions. If there is excessive give, an ACL injury is present. An anterior drawer test will also be positive. It is performed with the knee flexed to 90°. The examiner then sits on the foot of the ipsilateral extremity, places both hands behind the knee and attempts to pull it forward, like opening a drawer. If there is excessive give, an ACL injury is present;

ii) PCL [Figure 7]: injured if the patient has a positive posterior sag or posterior drawer test. This can easily be confused with a positive anterior drawer test. The posterior sag is the easiest way to differentiate. With the knee at 90° of flexion a pen or other straight item is laid along the anterior tibial crest up to the patella. Normally (try it on yourself) the pen stands away from the patella; if the posterior cruciate is deficient the tibia will sag backwards and the pen will lie on the patella. A posterior drawer test is performed in the same way as the anterior drawer test but the knee can be pulled

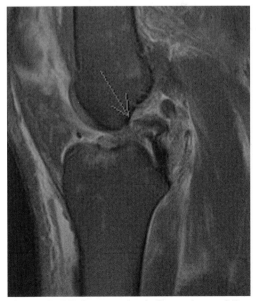

Figure 7. MR image depicting a tear of the PCL (arrow).

forward from the abnormal (sagging) to the normal position as opposed to moving from the normal to an abnormal anterior subluxated position;

iii) medial collateral ligament (MCL) and lateral collateral ligament (LCL) tear [Figures 8 and 9]: a varus and valgus stress test will identify excessive give when the knee is slightly flexed to relax the cruciate ligaments and the posterior capsule;

iv) posterolateral corner (PLC): the PLC is important in lateral knee stability, and is comprised of the popliteus tendon, LCL, and biceps femoris. To assess the integrity of the PLC all structures should be examined. LCL integrity is assessed by varus stress of the knee at 30° of flexion. The integrity of biceps femoris and the popliteus tendon [Figure 10] can be assessed by judging external rotation of the knee at 30° of flexion. If there is excessive rotation there is likely injury to these tendons.

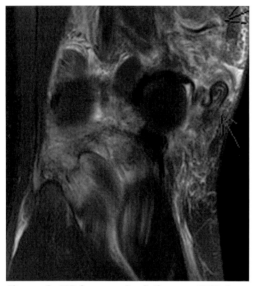

Figure 8. MR image depicting an MCL tear (arrow).

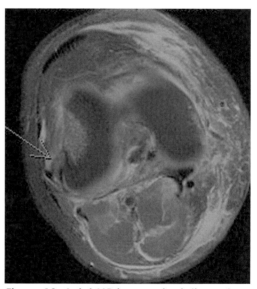

Figure 10. Axial MR image depicting a tear of the popliteus tendon.

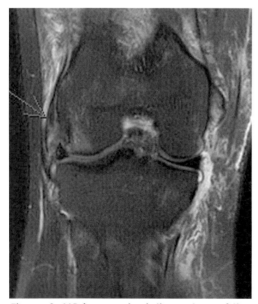

Figure 9. MR image depicting a tear of the LCL (fibular/lateral collateral ligament).

The amount of normal rotation and translation of a joint varies from patient to patient. For example, a gymnast or young child will have more laxity in their ligaments compared with the average adult. The best means of assessing if joint motion is abnormal with the above tests is to compare the amount of rotation/translation in the injured extremity to that of the non-injured extremity.

6. Low-energy knee dislocations occur in morbid obesity and should be considered with any presentation of acute knee pain in the morbidly obese. They typically occur after simply stepping off a curb and are commonly associated with a vascular injury. Because of the patient's size the dislocation may be invisible.

Management

Knee dislocations are an orthopedic emergency due to the tenuous neurovascular status of the injured extremity. Priority is given to vascular status first, and then to neurologic status. In this patient, the extremity is pulseless and needs to be reduced emergently. Waiting for conscious sedation is not necessary and the reduction should be performed in the trauma bay.

The method of reduction for anterior dislocation is to first apply axial traction to the tibia. This will pull it away from the femur. An assistant should then lift the distal femur to bring it in line with the tibia and reduce the joint.

Once the joint is reduced, pulses should be re-checked. If there are still no distal pulses, emergency vascular reconstruction is required. If pulses return, but are diminished, or the capillary refill is slow, or the ankle-brachial index (ABI) is less than 0.9, a vascular injury is still likely and an emergent angiography should be performed to evaluate for an intimal tear. If pulses return and are palpable, undiminished, with brisk capillary refill, and an ABI greater than 0.9, vascular injury is less likely but the patient should be observed for any sign of vascular compromise.

Should the patient have to go to the operating theater for vascular repair, then the extremity should be placed in an external fixator to maintain reduction and stability of the vasculature. If pulses return after reduction, the patient can be placed in a knee immobilizer to prevent movement of the joint and re-dislocation.

Once a vascular repair is performed, the patient also needs to be monitored carefully for reperfusion compartment syndrome. Prophylactic fasciotomies are recommended.

In an anterior dislocation, there is a greater likelihood of an intimal tear, and after posterior dislocation the patient is more likely to have a laceration of the popliteal artery; pulses may not return after reduction.

Once the patient's knee has been stabilized, an MRI can be performed to evaluate for ligamentous injury. These structures can be repaired early or delayed until some knee motion has been regained.

For neurologic compromise, simple bracing to prevent foot drop is used. In general, functional recovery is often poor.

Key points

- Knee dislocations are orthopedic emergencies.
- They are associated with neurovascular damage, of which the vascular injury should be treated as a major emergency.
- Anterior dislocations are the most common anatomic type, followed by posterior dislocations.
- These injuries should be reduced emergently, and careful attention paid to vascular status.
- Low-energy dislocations occur in the morbidly obese.

References

1. Shelbourne KD, Klootwyk TE. Low velocity knee dislocation with sports injuries: treatment principles. *Clin Sports Med* 2000; 19: 443-56.

2. Kennedy JC. Complete dislocation of the knee joint. *J Bone Joint Surg [Am]* 1963; 45: 889-904.

3. Kennedy JC, Hawkins RJ, Willis RB, *et al.* Tension studies of human ligaments: yield points, ultimate failure, and disruption of the cruciate and tibial collateral ligaments. *J Bone Joint Surg [Am]* 1976; 58: 350.

4. Koval KJ, Zuckerman JD. *Handbook of Fractures,* 3rd ed. Philadelphia, PA: Lippincott Williams & Wilkins, 2006.

Case 3

Clinical presentation

A 21-year-old field hockey player is hit by a ball on the lateral aspect of her left knee. She presents to the ER with pain and difficulty bearing weight on her left leg.

Physical examination

The skin is intact. There is swelling over the lateral knee but no gross effusion. The knee is stable to varus and valgus stress but varus stress is very painful. Range of motion of the knee is near full but limited by pain. There is tenderness localized over the fibular head. She has no foot drop, and sensation of the superficial peroneal nerve is intact.

Review the images below [Figures 11 and 12]. Describe your findings.

Questions

1. What is the diagnosis?

2. What does the arcuate complex consist of? What is the arcuate sign?

3. What is the mechanism of injury?

4. Why is this injury important?

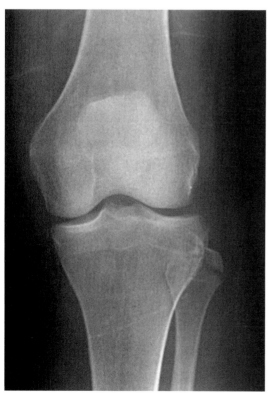

Figure 11.

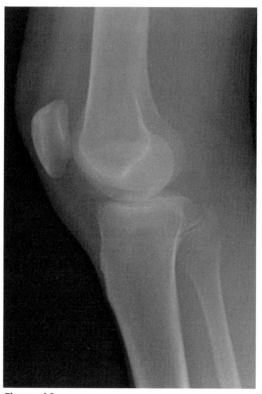

Figure 12.

Radiology findings

There is an avulsion fracture at the lateral base of the fibular head, known as the fibular styloid process. The long axis of the avulsion fracture is orientated in a horizontal plane on the frontal radiograph.

Answers

1. Avulsion fracture of the fibular head.

2. The arcuate complex consists of the fabellofibular, popliteofibular, and arcuate ligaments. A fibular head fracture can involve disruption of the arcuate complex and may be associated with posterolateral corner instability of the knee. The arcuate sign is synonymous with an avulsion fracture of the fibular head, and is important because it is often associated with posterolateral corner instability of the knee.

3. Typically, patients present with this injury after a direct blow to the anterior aspect of the extended knee.

4. This injury may be subtle and missed on initial examination. It is important because it may indicate posterolateral knee instability. Further evaluation with an MRI should be performed, to assess for concomitant damage to the PCL, collateral ligaments, and menisci. Other structures in the posterolateral corner of the knee may also be affected, such as the popliteal and biceps femoris tendons.

Management

In isolation, this injury is treated non-operatively. Most patients can weight bear as tolerated. If they are uncomfortable, they may be kept non-weight bearing with crutches and slowly progress to full weight bearing as comfort permits.

Key points

♦ An avulsion fracture of the fibular head often indicates posterolateral knee instability.

♦ The arcuate sign is an avulsion fracture of the fibular head.

♦ An MRI may be indicated to evaluate the posterolateral corner and the other intra-articular structures, especially if the patient's knee feels unstable on physical examination.

References

1. Shindell R, Walsh WM, Connolly JF. Avulsion fracture of the fibula: the 'arcuate sign' of posterolateral knee instability. *Nebra Med J* 1984; 69: 369-71.

2. Veltri DM, Warren RF. Posterolateral instability of the knee. *J Bone Joint Surg [Am]* 1994; 76: 460-72.

3. Huang GS, Yu JS, Munshi M, *et al.* Avulsion fracture of the head of the fibula (the 'arcuate sign'): MR imaging findings predictive of injuries to the posterolateral ligaments and posterior cruciate ligament. *AJR Am J Roentgenol* 2003; 180: 381-7.

4. Koval KJ, Zuckerman JD. *Handbook of Fractures*, 3rd ed. Philadelphia, PA: Lippincott Williams & Wilkins, 2006.

Case 4

Clinical presentation

A 48-year-old woman presents to the ER after a skiing injury. She was skiing downhill and fell. She reports that her right knee 'twisted inward' during her fall. She presents with pain and difficulty ambulating.

Physical examination

On physical exam, the patient has a slight knee effusion. The skin is intact, and there is no ecchymosis. The patient has pain with a range of motion of the knee, and pain with valgus stress. She splints with valgus stress, making it difficult to determine instability. She has tenderness over the medial and lateral joint lines, and a positive anterior drawer test and a negative posterior drawer test. Due to discomfort, a pivot shift test and Lachman's test are deferred.

Review the image below [Figure 13]. Describe your findings.

Questions

1. What is the diagnosis?

2. What is the mechanism of injury?

3. What other associated injuries may be present?

4. What is involved in the reverse version of this injury?

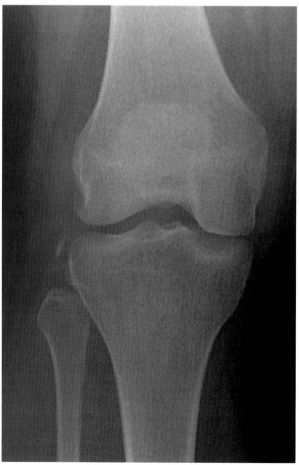

Figure 13.

Radiology findings

An anteroposterior radiograph demonstrates an avulsion fracture of the lateral aspect of the proximal tibia, slightly below the articular surface. The fragment is elliptical and separated from the tibia by a vertical fracture line. An MRI further depicts this avulsion fracture with marrow edema in the proximal tibia and distal femur [Figure 14]. On the sagittal image, the ACL is torn [Figure 15].

Answers

1. Segond fracture.

2. A Segond fracture occurs due to internal rotation and varus stress. This results in abnormal tension on the central portion of the iliotibial band or anterior oblique band of the LCL of the knee, which can cause an avulsion fracture of the lateral proximal tibia.

3. Other injuries that can be present include disruption of the ACL (seen in 75-100% of cases), lateral and medial meniscal injuries (seen in 66-75% of cases), and avulsion fractures of the fibular head and/or Gerdy's tubercle (insertion of the iliotibial band).

4. A 'reverse Segond' fracture is an avulsion of the deep MCL and may be associated with disruption of the PCL and a peripheral medial meniscal tear. On plain films, this injury is visualized as a small bone fragment adjacent to the medial tibial plateau.

Management

An important aspect of these fractures is recognizing the associated ligamentous and meniscal injuries. An isolated avulsion fracture that is not symptomatic to the patient can be treated non-operatively. However, if there are associated lateral meniscal and ACL injuries, these may require staged

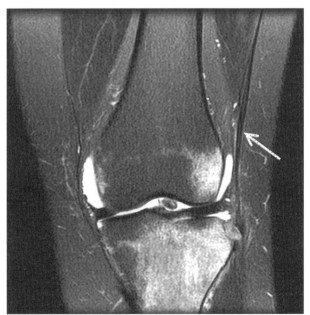

Figure 14. Coronal T2 fat saturated-weighted image demonstrating an avulsion fracture at the lateral aspect of the proximal tibia, with marrow edema within both the femur and tibia. The fragment is attached to the iliotibial band (arrow).

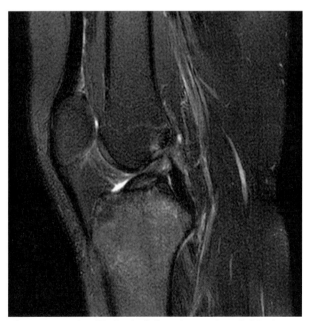

Figure 15. Sagittal T2 fat saturated-weighted MR image shows disruption of the ACL.

operative fixation. Therefore, when a Segond fracture is identified, an MRI should be performed to evaluate the ACL, and lateral meniscus. If these are not injured, and there are no findings on physical exam to suggest such injuries, the patient can be placed in a knee immobilizer and given crutches, and allowed to weight bear as tolerated. If there is an associated ACL and/or medial meniscal injury, the patient may have the same initial management but will need surgical fixation of the associated injuries. The Segond fracture may be treated by screw fixation when the ACL is reconstructed.

Key points

- A Segond fracture is an avulsion fracture of the lateral aspect of the proximal tibia below the articular surface.

- It involves the insertion of the iliotibial band or anterior oblique band of the fibular collateral ligament.

- There is a high incidence of associated disruption of the ACL, best seen on an MRI.

- These injuries are important to identify due to the possibility of associated lateral meniscal and ACL injuries.

References

1. Capps GW, Hayes CW. Easily missed injuries around the knee. *Radiographic* 1994; 14: 1191-210.

2. Dietz GW, Wilcox DM, Montgomery JB. Segond tibial condyle fracture: lateral capsular ligament avulsion. *Radiology* 1986; 159: 467-9.

3. Goldman AB, Pavlow H, Rubenstein D. The Segond fracture of the proximal tibia: a small avulsion that reflects major ligamentous damage. *AJR Am J Roentgenol* 1988; 151: 1163-7.

4. Rogers LF. The knee and shafts of the tibia and fibula. *In: Radiology of Skeletal Trauma*, Vol 2, 2nd ed. New York, NY: Churchill Livingstone, 1992: 1199-317.

5. Escobedo EM, Mills WJ, Hunter JC. The 'reverse Segond' fracture: association with a tear of the posterior cruciate ligament and medial meniscus. *AJR Am J Roentgenol* 2002; 178(4): 979-83.

6. Segond P. Recherches cliniques et expérimentales sur les épanchements sanguins du genou par entorse. *Progres Med* 1879; 7: 297-9, 319-21, 340-1.

Case 5

Clinical presentation

A 42-year-old male presents after being struck at low speed by a vehicle bumper while crossing the street. He presents with an isolated injury to the left knee. There are no other injuries or complaints. He reports diffuse left knee pain and cannot walk.

Physical examination

The skin is intact, and there is diffuse swelling with an effusion in the knee and tenderness over the lateral aspect of the knee. The knee is too painful to assess varus and valgus instability. The distal circulation is intact with palpable foot pulses. Distal sensation and motor function is intact. The lower leg compartments are soft and compressible.

Review the images below [Figures 16 and 17]. Describe your findings.

Questions

1. What is the diagnosis?

2. What other associated injuries can occur?

3. What is the most common classification system used? Describe it.

4. What types of mechanisms of injury can result in this injury?

5. List the long-term complications which may occur as a result of this injury.

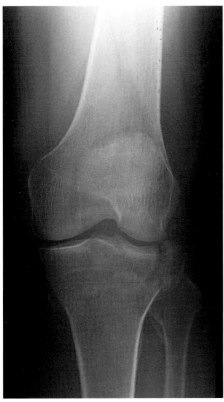

Figure 16.

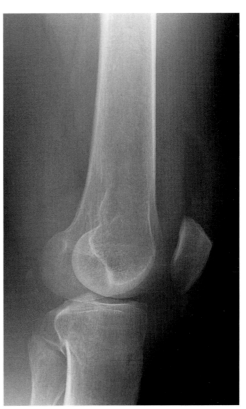

Figure 17.

Radiology findings

There is a comminuted, split fracture of the lateral tibial plateau, with depression of the plateau. The fracture plane extends into the tibial metaphysis and exits through the medial metaphysis. On the lateral image, a lipohemarthrosis is seen. CT images are usually obtained to further characterize the degree of plateau depression and fragmentation [Figures 18 and 19]. It is useful for pre-operative planning and important as plain films can under-estimate the degree of involvement. In addition, it also gives information about associated tendinous and ligamentous injuries.

Answers

1. Lateral tibial plateau fracture Type VI.

2. A variety of remote and local associated injuries can occur with tibial plateau fractures, and depend on the extent of the fracture and mechanism of injury. The mechanism is often associated with more serious, even life-threatening remote injuries which must be excluded. Tibial plateau fractures can also be associated with neurovascular compromise to the limb if the peroneal nerve or popliteal vessels are injured. When an axial loading mechanism is involved, calcaneal [Figure 20] and spinal fractures should be specifically looked for. Locally, compartment syndrome is uncommon but very important. It can occur especially if the injury involved high energy. The

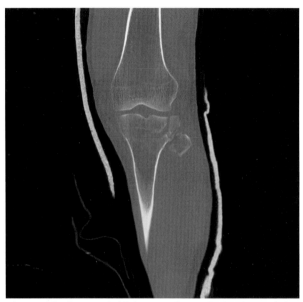

Figure 18. Coronal CT image through the knee joint depicts a Schatzker Type VI injury. An associated fibular head fracture is also noted.

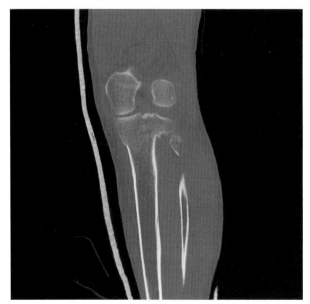

Figure 19. Coronal CT image through the knee further depicts the injury seen in Figure 18.

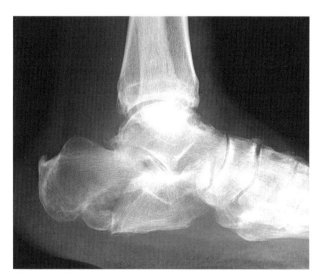

Figure 20. A lateral radiograph of the foot demonstrates a comminuted calcaneal fracture in this patient after high-energy trauma. The patient was also found to have a fracture of the lateral tibial plateau (not shown).

menisci collateral and cruciate ligaments can also be injured. Examination in the acute phase may not be valuable and MRI may be considered. The further the lateral plateau is displaced laterally, the more likely there is a peripheral detachment of the lateral meniscus.

3. The Schatzker classification system is the most widely used for tibial plateau fractures and incorporates both medial and lateral fractures [Figure 21]:
   i) Type I fractures are split fractures of the lateral plateau and are associated with a high incidence of MCL injuries [Figures 22 and 23]. There may be an associated lateral meniscal tear;
   ii) Type II fractures are split fractures of the lateral plateau with depression of a central fragment of the plateau. There may be associated damage to the lateral meniscus, medial meniscus, and/or MCL;

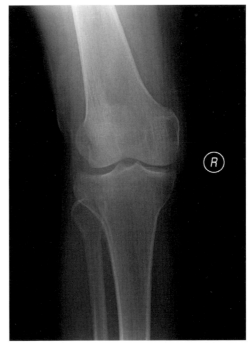

Figure 22. AP radiograph demonstrates a fracture of the lateral tibial plateau without significant depression or displacement of fragments, classified as a Schatzker Type I injury.

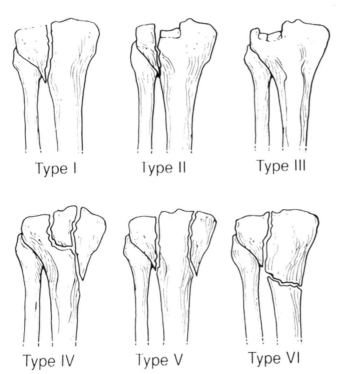

Type I   Type II   Type III

Type IV   Type V   Type VI

Figure 21. Schatzker's classification of tibial plateau fractures. *Reprinted with permission from Thieme Publishers, © 1979. From Schatzker J, McBroom R, Bruce D. The tibial plateau fracture. The Toronto experience 1968-1975. Clin Orthop Relat Res 1979; 138: 94.*

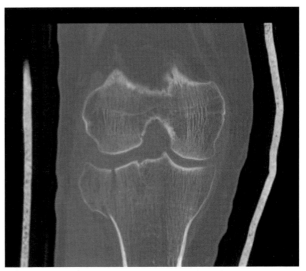

Figure 23. A coronal CT image further characterizes the degree of involvement of the fracture.

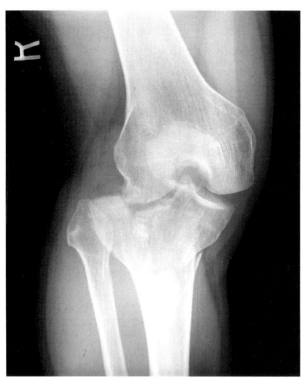

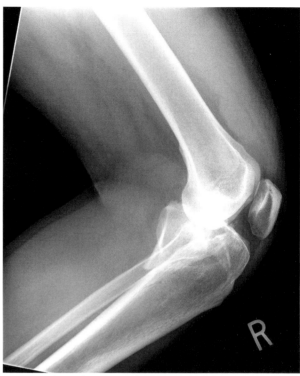

Figure 24. AP and lateral radiographs of the right knee demonstrate a fracture dislocation of the knee with a Schatzker Type IV fracture of the medial tibial plateau.

iii) Type III fractures involve depressions of the whole lateral plateau fracture and may be associated with joint instability;

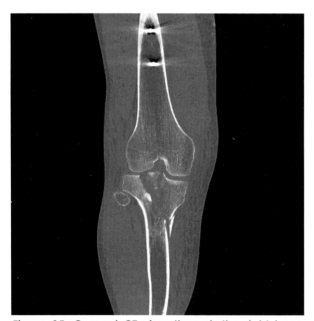

Figure 25. Coronal CT view through the right knee confirms a Schatzker Type IV injury.

iv) Type IV injuries are fracture dislocations of the knee with a medial plateau fracture [Figures 24 and 25]. They are high-energy injuries and are frequently associated with damage to other adjacent structures such as the popliteal artery, peroneal nerve, LCL and the medial meniscus. An avulsion of the intercondylar eminence will indicate a cruciate ligament injury;

v) Type V injuries are bicondylar plateau fractures with intact tibial spines and can result in compartment syndrome. There may also be neurovascular, ACL, and meniscal injuries;

vi) Type VI is a bicondylar fracture that results in separation of the tibial metaphysis from the diaphysis. The fracture is typically comminuted and can result in compartment syndrome. Other associated injuries include neurovascular injury, and meniscal, ACL, and collateral ligament injuries.

Tibial plateau fractures can also be classified by the OTA/AO system as 'A', 'B' and 'C' type injuries.

4. Tibial plateau fractures are most often seen after significant trauma with a blow on the side of the knee such as vehicle bumper injuries. Other mechanisms including sports and falls are common.

5. Complications relate to the adequacy of articular reduction at healing and associated injuries. There may be knee stiffness and post-traumatic osteoarthritis. Malunion or non-union may result and are more common with Schatzker Type VI fractures. Infection after surgery is rare but it is important to recognise and treat any infection accordingly.

Management

In general, while non-displaced, stable fractures can be treated non-operatively, displaced or unstable fractures need operative reduction and stabilization. The aim is to provide anatomical reduction of the joint surface and allow early motion to provide normal function in the long term.

Non-operative treatment:

♦ Non-displaced fracture. Initially the knee will be immobilized and the patient made non-weight bearing on crutches. Usually, this will be rapidly converted to a hinged knee brace, providing a free range of motion but varus/valgus stability and the patient allowed to touch down weight bear until the fracture is healed, normally at 8-12 weeks. More aggressive therapy and weight bearing will begin as the fracture heals.

Operative management:

♦ Displaced, unstable fractures need operative reduction and internal fixation. Rarely, external fixation may be used either temporarily or for definitive fracture management. If there is doubt about the stability, examination under anesthesia may be used to assess any varus or valgus instability.
♦ Operative stabilization is indicated:
   i) if there is more than 10° of instability with the leg in extension as compared with the non-injured extremity;
   ii) if there is loss of fracture position in follow-up;

iii) if the patient presents with complications such as compartment syndrome, open fractures or those with vascular compromise.

A general review of tibial plateau fracture management is as follows:

♦ Type I: open reduction and internal fixation (ORIF) with a lag screw/plate fixation.
♦ Type II: ORIF with elevation of depressed fragments (either through open arthrotomy or a smaller cortical window), with a lag screw/plate fixation.
♦ Type III: often non-operative management in the elderly if the fracture is stable to varus and valgus stress.
♦ Type IV: ORIF with a medial buttress plate to stabilize against shear force against the medial side of the knee.
♦ Type V: ORIF often with a buttress plate on both medial and lateral sides.
♦ Type VI: ORIF with joint reconstruction with lag screws followed by stabilization of the joint block to the tibial diaphysis with a laterally placed locking plate. Bilateral plates or a definitive external fixator may be used.

Key points

♦ A tibial plateau fracture is an intra-articular fracture of the proximal tibia.
♦ Lateral tibial plateau fractures are more common than medial plateau fractures and are often associated with meniscal or ligamentous injury.
♦ CT imaging with axial reformats is used to assess the extent of the fracture and to plan surgical management.
♦ More unstable fracture patterns are seen in younger patients.
♦ There are four main features of a fracture that will help to classify the injury and select an appropriate method of treatment. These include classification, displacement, stability and associated soft tissue injury.

References

1. Schatzker J, McBroom R, Bruce D. The tibial plateau fracture. The Toronto experience 1968-1975. *Clin Orthop Relat Res* 1979; (138): 94-104.

2. Walton NP, Harish S, Roberts C, Blundell C. AO or Schatzker? How reliable is classification of tibial plateau fractures? *Arch Orthop Trauma Surg* 2003; 123(8): 396-8.

3. Gardner MJ, Yacoubian S, Geller D, Pode D, Mintz D, Helfet DL. Prediction of soft tissue injuries in Schatzker II tibial plateau fractures based on measurements of plain radiographs. *Journal of Trauma* 2006; 60(2): 319-24.

4. Tigges S, Fajman WA. Injuries about the knee and tibial/fibular shafts. *Semin Musculoskelet Radiol* 2000; 4(2): 221-39.

5. Anglen JO, Healy WL. Tibial plateau fractures. *Orthopedics* 1988; 11(11): 1527-34.

6. Barrow BA, Fajman WA, Parker LM, *et al.* Tibial plateau fractures: evaluation with MR imaging. *Radiographics* 1994; 14(3): 553-9.

Case 6

Clinical presentation

A 53-year-old man presents to the ER after having his leg pinned between the bumpers of two cars. He had been crossing the street between two parked cars when one vehicle reversed, pinning the patient's leg between the reversing vehicle and the stationary one immediately behind it. There are no other injuries.

Physical examination

There is gross swelling of the proximal to mid-tibia. The skin has abrasions over the area of direct contact, but no open injury. The leg feels swollen and tight, but distally there is a palpable dorsalis pedis pulse. He is too uncomfortable to adequately answer questions about sensation in his foot. He has pain with passive range of motion of his toes.

Review the images below [Figures 26 and 27]. Describe your findings.

Questions

1. What is the diagnosis?

2. What is the mechanism of injury?

3. What are some identifiers for compartment syndrome?

4. Describe the Tscherne classification system, and how this fracture fits into it.

5. Describe the blood supply to the tibia. Why is this important?

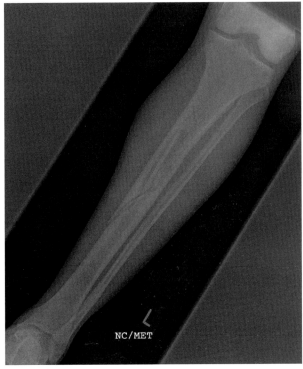

Figure 26.

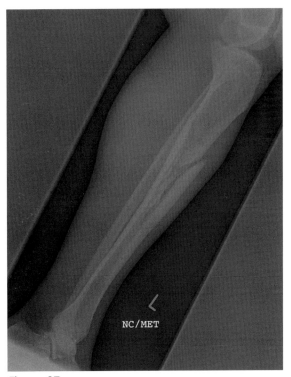

Figure 27.

Radiology findings

AP and lateral radiographs of the tibia and fibula show a midshaft, comminuted fracture of the tibia.

Answers

1. Comminuted tibial shaft fracture with likely compartment syndrome.

2. This is a crush injury. Other typical mechanisms include motor vehicle accidents and injuries during sports or falls. Fracture patterns correspond to the force applied and the degree of destruction to the energy applied. In crush injuries (as well as other tibial fractures), the soft tissue element of the injury often dominates the clinical picture.

3. Compartment syndrome should be suspected clinically. Pain out of proportion to the injury or examination, or pain with passive motion of toes/fingers, can be helpful indicators of lower and upper extremity compartment syndrome. Objective measurement involves direct measurement of compartment pressure where a differential of >30mm Hg below diastolic pressure is considered diagnostic and an indication for surgical release (unless the patient is hypotensive). There are four compartments in the lower leg: the anterior, superficial posterior, deep posterior and lateral compartments. All these should be released if a fasciotomy is performed.

4. This is most likely a Tscherne Grade III fracture due to compartment syndrome. This classification system for closed fractures is as follows:
    i)   Grade 0: indirect force causing low-energy injury. Little to no soft tissue damage (torsional fracture or a stress fracture may fall into this category);
    ii) Grade I: closed fracture. Low to moderate-energy injury. Superficial abrasions with minor underlying muscle contusion;
    iii) Grade II: closed fracture. Moderate to severe-energy injury. Deep abrasions with significant underlying muscle contusion and possible compartment syndrome;
    iv) Grade III: closed fracture. Crushing injury. Significant underlying muscle contusion, arterial disruption and compartment syndrome.

5. The posterior tibial artery gives rise to a nutrient artery which enters the posterolateral tibial cortex and gives off three ascending branches and two descending branches in the canal. These anastomose with periosteal vessels from the anterior tibial artery. This is important because a large part of the tibial blood supply comes from the periosteum. In fracture fixation, especially when there is found to be a disruption of the posterior tibial artery, it is important not to overly strip the periosteum in order to preserve blood supply and promote healing.

Management

In this patient there is a clinical compartment syndrome. This is a surgical emergency. The patient should be taken emergently to the operating theater and a full fasciotomy should be performed. Any major vascular injury should be dealt with appropriately. Surgical fracture stabilization should be performed. The method will be chosen based on the fracture anatomy and the condition of the local soft tissues. Since the patient is so swollen, with significant soft tissue damage, it may be reasonable to initially place him in an external fixator until his swelling decreases and his fasciotomy wounds can be closed. At that time, an intramedullary nail can be used for definitive internal fixation.

Not all tibial shaft fractures need operative fixation. In those that are minimally displaced and remain in a good position, non-operative care in a plaster cast and, subsequently, a tibial brace may be very successful.

Key points

- In high-energy tibial shaft fractures and very comminuted fractures, be wary of compartment syndrome.
- A large part of the tibial blood supply is periosteal.
- Beware compartment syndrome if the pain is out of proportion to the situation. Measurement of compartment pressures is definitive if the differential between the compartment pressure and diastolic pressure is less than 30mm Hg.

References

1. McQueen MM, Court-Brown CM. Compartment monitoring in tibial fractures. The pressure threshold for decompression. *J Bone Joint Surg [Br]* 1996; 78(1): 99-104

Chapter 8

Ankle and foot

Case 1

Clinical presentation

A 42-year-old woman steps off a curb in her high heels and twists her ankle outwards. She hears a 'pop', feels immediate pain, and is unable to bear weight. She notes immediate swelling and deformity of her ankle, and presents to the ER for further evaluation.

Physical examination

Grossly, the skin is intact and there is swelling and ecchymosis of the ankle. There is tenderness to palpation over the medial and lateral malleoli. The patient will not plantar or dorsiflex her ankle secondary to pain. She will, however, flex and extend her toes with some discomfort. She reports good sensation in her ankle and foot. She has a palpable dorsalis pedis pulse, and Doppler is used to detect the posterior tibial pulse secondary to swelling. A strong triphasic waveform is heard on Doppler.

Review the image below [Figure 1]. Describe your findings.

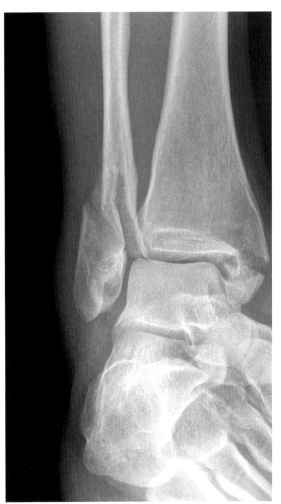

Figure 1.

Questions

1. What is the diagnosis?

2. What is the mechanism of injury?

3. How are ankle fractures classified?

4. What are important radiographic findings to observe when evaluating the ankle?

5. Describe the ligamentous anatomy of the ankle.

Radiology findings

An oblique comminuted acute fracture at the distal fibula at the level of the tibial plafond is seen with mild lateral displacement of the dominant distal fracture fragment. Also noted is a comminuted transverse fracture at the medial malleolus. There is inferior distraction of the distal fracture fragment over a maximal 6mm distance. There is lateral subluxation of the talus. Mild lateral shift of the ankle mortise is seen.

Answers

1. Weber Type B ankle fracture with a medial malleolar fracture.

2. Weber Type B fractures occur due to the application of external rotation and abduction to the ankle. A rotational fracture occurs in the fibula followed by an avulsion of the medial malleolus. If the force continues the avulsion will create a transverse fracture on the medial side as opposed to the oblique fracture laterally. Instability is judged by displacement but these are often unstable and require operative stabilization.

3. The Weber classification is used for ankle fractures, and specifically considers the fibula as this relates to the principal mode of stability of the ankle. The fractures are considered as A, B and C types [Figure 2] according to the height of the lateral fracture and, by implication, the involvement of the distal tibiofibular ligament complex:

   i) in Weber A fractures, there is a transverse fracture of the lateral malleolus distal to the syndesmotic ligaments with or without a vertical or oblique fracture of the medial malleolus [Figure 3]. This represents the opposite mechanism with a push-off vertical fracture of the medial malleolus and avulsion

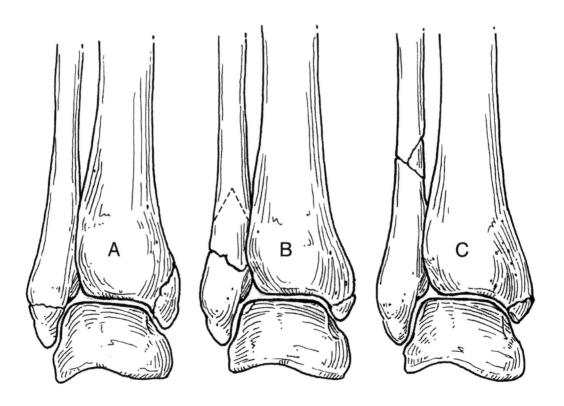

Figure 2. The Weber classification for ankle fractures. *Reprinted with permission from the Radiological Society of North America. Hunter T, Peltier L, Lund P, et al. Musculoskeletal eponyms: who are those guys? Radiographics 2000; 20(3): 819-36.*

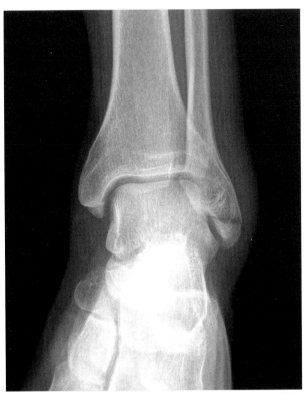

Figure 3. Frontal radiograph of the right ankle demonstrates a transverse lateral malleolar fracture (Weber A) with good alignment and apposition of the fracture fragments. There is no lateral talar tilt or displacement. The medial malleolus is intact. This is an avulsion injury of the fibula distal to the syndesmotic ligaments. This is equivalent to the Lauge-Hansen stage I injury named supination-adduction (SA).

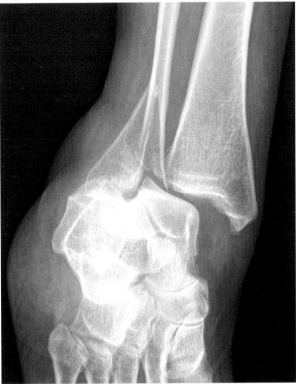

Figure 4. There is an oblique fracture through the distal fibula at the level of the syndesmosis with displacement of the distal fracture fragments and anterolateral subluxation of the distal tibia. There are no fractures of the talus and medial malleolus. There is clear talar shift and the tibiofibular space is widened (greater than 5mm). There is a lateral talar tilt and widening of the ankle mortise. This is consistent with a Weber Type B injury with lateral dislocation at the ankle joint.

of the tip of the fibula. By implication the tibiofibular ligaments are spared but an impaction fracture of the medial tibial plafond surface may also be present. This is equivalent to the Lauge-Hansen supination-adduction injury;

ii) in Weber Type B fractures, there is a fracture of the fibula beginning at the level of the tibial plafond, at or near the level of the syndesmosis [Figure 4]. It typically extends proximally and posteriorly through the fibular shaft. The posterior syndesmotic ligament usually remains intact. This is equivalent to the Lauge-Hansen supination-eversion injury;

iii) in Weber Type C fractures, the fracture line is above the syndesmosis. The posterior malleolus may be avulsed with the unstable fibula fragment due to the intact ligament that holds both fragments. The medial injury represents an avulsion of the bone or ligamentous complex medially. The orientation of a fracture line is transverse representing the avulsion of the medial malleolus. The syndesmosis is always involved. This is equivalent to the Lauge-Hansen supination-external rotation injury. This type of fracture is usually very unstable, and requires reduction and surgical stabilization.

4. When evaluating ankle films for a fracture, there are certain areas to assess. The joint space around the talus should be the same all around the bone on the mortise view. An increase on either side implies talar shift and instability. For example, if the medial clear space is greater than the lateral clear space of the superior ankle joint, this indicates a lateral talar tilt. The talocrural angle is also an important finding. This angle is obtained by drawing a line between the tips of the medial and lateral malleoli (intermalleollar line) and a line parallel to the distal tibial articular surface on the mortise view. This angle is usually 8-15° in a normal ankle and will be greater if displaced by injury. Fibular shortening is present if this angle is 2-5° greater than that of the opposite side. On a mortise view, the tibiofibular line is that formed between the distal tibia and medial aspect of the fibula. It should be continuous with the lateral articular surface of the talus and if disrupted, indicates shortening, lateral displacement and external rotation of the fibula. The distal tibia and fibula normally have an overlap of 1cm. Less than 1cm of overlap indicates syndesmotic injury. Finally, the lateral view should be assessed for posterior malleolar fractures or anterior talar avulsion fractures.

5. The ligaments around the ankle syndesmosis help to maintain stability and alignment of the ankle joint. These ligaments include the syndesmotic ligament complex, the deltoid ligament complex, and the fibular collateral ligament complex:

i) the syndesmotic complex includes the inferior tibiofibular ligament, the posterior inferior tibiofibular ligament, and the transverse tibiofibular ligament. The posterior inferior tibiofibular ligament is the strongest of the three. The transverse tibiofibular ligament is located inferior to the posterior tibiofibular ligament. The interosseous ligament is also part of the complex;

ii) the deltoid ligament complex supports the medial joint, and is made up of superficial and deep components. The superficial components include the tibionavicular ligament (prevents inward talar displacement), the tibio-calcaneal ligament (prevents valgus displacement), and the superficial tibiotalar ligament. The deep component includes the deep tibiotalar ligament, which is the primary medial stabilizer of the ankle;

iii) the fibular collateral ligament is made of three ligaments. These include the anterior talofibular ligament (weakest of the three, prevents anterior talar subluxation when the foot is plantar flexed), the posterior talofibular ligament (strongest of the three, prevents rotary and posterior talar subluxation), and lastly, there is the calcaneofibular ligament, which limits talar inversion.

Management

A non-displaced or stable fracture pattern, such as a Weber Type A fracture, that does not involve the syndesmosis, or that results in a stable syndesmotic injury, can be treated non-operatively. These patients can be placed in an aircast boot and allowed to be weight bearing as tolerated. Any non-displaced fracture or those, such as Weber Type B or C injuries, in which a stable anatomic reduction is obtained, can be placed in a U-splint. When swelling has decreased these patients can be placed in a cast and kept non-weight bearing until evidence of healing. Most Weber Type B and C fractures, however, are unstable, and need operative intervention to maintain reduction. As a result most of these fractures are treated by open reduction and internal fixation (ORIF) following AO principles.

The initial reduction performed in the emergency room can be done using a local intra-articular injection, or with conscious sedation. The goal is to take the stress off the skin and realign the mortise. An assistant holds the patient's knee flexed to relax the gastrocnemius-soleus complex. The surgeon stands at the foot of the table. For the injury above, the talus needs to be brought back medially. One hand is placed over the distal tibia, and the other hand on the lateral malleolus. Pressure is applied in opposite directions, with force directed in the medial direction with the hand over the lateral malleolus, and counter-traction applied using the hand over the distal tibial shaft. The mortise is held reduced using the Quigley maneuver (applying traction to the great toe of the injured extremity), while a U-splint with a posterior slab is applied to the ankle. The right leg should then be iced and elevated on two pillows to keep swelling at a minimum

The principal issue to consider is the nature of the soft tissue injury. If there is too much swelling, or fracture blisters, the soft tissues should be allowed time to heal before surgical correction is considered. Normally at surgery, the fibula is fixed first. The common, simple oblique fracture is fixed anatomically with absolute stability using a lag screw and a neutralization plate across the fracture site. A typical transverse medial fracture is stabilized with two partially threaded lag screws. If the mortise is then stable on stress testing, additional diastasis screws (between the tibia and fibula) are not required. If the mortise is unstable on stress testing diastasis screws are inserted with the fibula anatomically reduced in its fossa on the lateral side of the tibia. The patient's weight bearing status is determined based on the stability of fixation, and the surgeon's own particular practice.

Key points

- Weber Type B ankle fractures involve the distal fibula at the level of the tibial plafond in the region of the syndesmosis.
- In nearly 50% of cases, the anterior syndesmotic ligament is partially or completely torn, but the posterior syndesmotic ligament usually remains intact.
- Weber Type A ankle fractures are distal to the mortise, and are usually stable injuries.
- Operative versus non-operative intervention depends on the reduction and its stability. At surgery, the fibula is usually reduced first, followed by the medial malleolus if required. Additional fixation between the tibia and fibula depends on the stability of the mortise.

References

1. Hunter T, Peltier L, Lund P. Musculoskeletal eponyms: who are those guys? *Radiographics* 2000; 20(3): 819-36.
2. Koval KJ, Zuckerman JD. *Handbook of Fractures*, 3rd ed. Philadelphia, PA: Lippincott Williams & Wilkins, 2006.

Case 2

Clinical presentation

A 43-year-old construction worker falls off the scaffolding, landing on his feet. He has no loss of consciousness, and no head injury. He presents to the ER for further evaluation. The team begins a full trauma survey of the patient. An orthopedic consult is called to evaluate the left lower extremity.

Physical examination

The patient is only injured around the left lower leg which is swollen and painful. There is diffuse ecchymosis around the ankle but the skin is intact. The patient has pain with palpation of the medial and lateral malleoli, and will not allow any ankle or subtalar range of motion. His sensation is intact in the foot and ankle. The pulses are not palpable due to swelling but the toes appear viable. With Doppler ultrasound, a biphasic wave is heard for both the dorsalis pedis and posterior tibial pulses.

Review the images below [Figures 5 and 6]. Describe your findings.

Questions

1. What is the diagnosis?

2. What is the mechanism of injury?

3. How are these injuries classified?

4. What is the main factor that determines timing of fixation of the fracture?

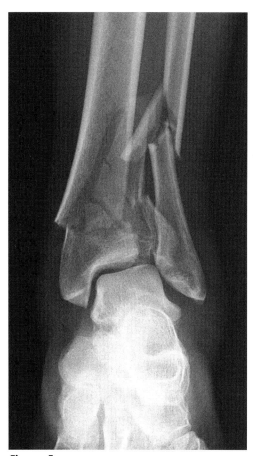

Figure 5.

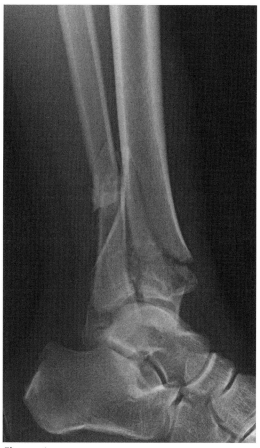

Figure 6.

Radiology findings

There is a comminuted fracture of the distal tibial metaphysis, with the fracture extending to involve the articular surface of the tibiotalar joint. The primary fracture line is oblique and is orientated lateral to medial, originating at the tibial metaphysis. There is involvement of both the medial malleolus and the posterior tibial rim. The degree of comminution is better demonstrated on subsequent CT images [Figures 7-9}. CT imaging also demonstrates entrapment of the posterior tibial tendon [Figures 10 and 11].

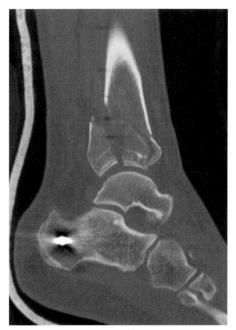

Figure 8. Sagittal CT image through the distal tibia and fibula confirms comminution of the distal tibia and involvement of the posterior tibial rim.

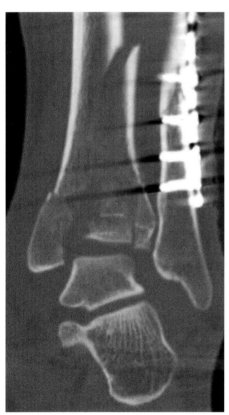

Figure 7. Coronal reformatted CT image demonstrates a comminuted fracture of the distal tibia. The patient is post-ORIF of a prior distal fibular fracture.

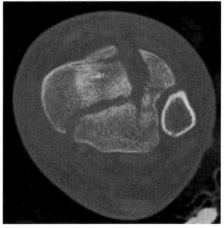

Figure 9. Axial CT image further delineates the degree of comminution.

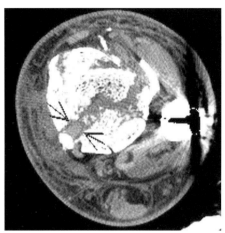

Figure 10. Axial CT image in soft tissue windows identifies the posterior tibial tendon entrapped within the fracture fragments (arrows).

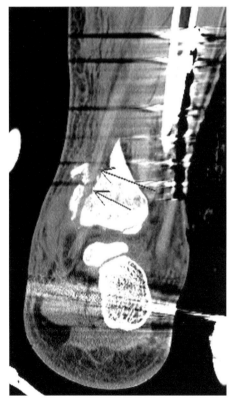

Figure 11. CT imaging is a useful modality for diagnosis of associated tendon or ligament pathology, demonstrating posterior tibial tendon entrapment in this patient.

Answers

1. Pilon fracture.

2. Pilon fractures are usually high-energy compression injuries, mostly following a fall from a height. The patient lands with their foot on the ground and the energy is transferred from the calcaneus to the talus. The talus impacts the distal tibia causing the fracture. The injury commonly includes metaphyseal and articular elements with varying degrees of comminution. Most commonly, the worst bone destruction is in the metaphyseal area. A variety of partial or complete articular fracture patterns can occur.

3. Pilon fractures are commonly divided into three types but more detailed classifications can also be used:
   i) Type I: intra-articular fracture without significant displacement of fracture fragments;
   ii) Type II: intra-articular, mildly comminuted fracture with disruption of the articular surface;
   iii) Type III: severely comminuted fracture with severe incongruity of the articular surface.

4. Pilon fractures are high-energy injuries. Due to this, damage to surrounding soft tissues and bone is often significant with swelling, bruising and development of fracture blisters because of occult soft tissue degloving. The anterior tibia is subcutaneous and, hence, open injuries are common. Early ORIF in the case of compromised, swollen soft tissues can lead to a higher rate of wound breakdown and subsequent infection. Commonly, definitive fixation is delayed until the soft tissues improve. An external fixator may be applied to support the fracture during this period.

Management

Non-displaced fractures can be treated non-operatively with early range of motion but non-weight bearing. Displaced intra-articular fractures are treated operatively. Initially, if the condition of the soft tissues will not allow early surgery, the patient is placed in an external fixator until the swelling decreases. The fracture is reduced closed as much as possible before the external fixator is placed. The patient is then later brought back for operative fixation. At formal reconstruction, the articular surface is reduced anatomically and metaphyseal defects traditionally bone grafted. There has been a move to percutaneous minimal invasive approaches (minimally invasive percutaneous plate osteosynthesis [MIPPO]) to limit the soft tissue and bony insult.

Key points

♦ Pilon fractures are high-energy injuries, with significant soft tissue damage.

♦ Quality of soft tissues often dictates timing of surgery.

♦ Due to the nature of these injuries, a full trauma workup is often performed, and associated injuries are searched for. Common associated injuries include calcaneal fractures, lumbar spine fractures, and tibial plateau fractures.

♦ These patients are often admitted for soft tissue management prior to surgery. Frequent neurovascular checks should be performed due to the extensive swelling, and patients should be monitored closely for compartment syndrome or soft tissue breakdown.

References

1. Tornetta P 3rd, Gorup J. Axial computed tomography of pilon fractures. *Clin Orthop* 1996; (323): 273-6.

2. Helfet DL, Koval K, Pappas J, Sanders RW, DiPasquale T. Intraarticular 'pilon' fracture of the tibia. *Clin Orthop* 1994; (298): 221-8.

3. Thordarson DB. Complications after treatment of tibial pilon fractures: prevention and management strategies. *J Am Acad Orthop Surg* 2000; 8(4): 253-65

4. Sirkin M, Sanders R. The treatment of pilon fractures. *Orthop Clin North Am* 2001; 32(1): 91-102.

5. Panchbhavi VK. Minimally invasive stabilization of pilon fractures. *Techniques in Foot and Ankle Surgery* 2005; 4 (4): 240-8.

6. Brumback RJ, McGarvey WC. Fractures of the tibial plafond. Evolving treatment concepts for the pilon fracture. *Orthop Clin North Am* 1995; 26(2): 273-85.

Case 3

Clinical presentation

A 30-year-old thief is running away from the police. He hops onto his getaway motorcycle, and during the chase, skids, and is thrown off his bike. He twists his foot during his crash and notices something white on the outside of his leg as he experiences excruciating pain. He presents to the ER in handcuffs and a wrap around his foot. He is unable to bear weight. He was a helmeted driver and had no loss of consciousness or head injury. However, he does have bruising as well as scrapes on his hands and elbows as he tried to break his fall. He is found to have an isolated foot injury.

Physical examination

There is bone extruding from the lateral aspect of the foot. The distal tibia and calcaneus are visible through the opening in the skin. There is swelling and surrounding ecchymosis. Distally, the patient has palpable dorsalis pedis and posterior tibial pulses. He reports intact sensation at the tips of his toes, but is in too much pain to fully co-operate with the motor exam.

Review the images below [Figures 12 and 13]. Describe your findings.

Questions

1. What is the diagnosis?

2. What is the mechanism of injury?

3. What complications may arise?

4. What is a total talar dislocation?

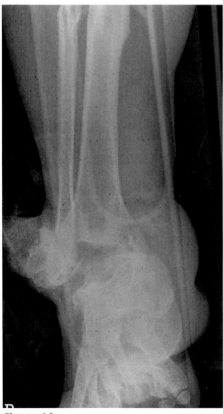

Figure 12.

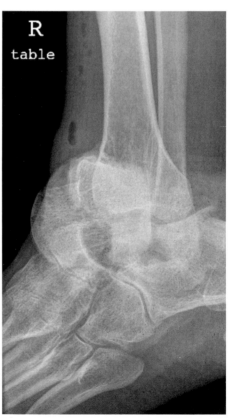

Figure 13.

Radiology findings

AP and lateral radiographs of the foot show a laterally dislocated talus, extruding out of the foot. There is dislocation of the tibiotalar, talonavicular, and talocalcaneal joints.

Answers

1. Medial talar dislocation.

2. Subtalar dislocations (also referred to as peritalar dislocations) are caused by both high-energy (motor vehicle accidents, fall from height) and low-energy mechanisms (sporting injuries, especially involving basketball). There are two main types of dislocations: medial and lateral. A medial subtalar dislocation occurs due to an inversion injury (most common) and results in medial displacement of the calcaneus and lateral displacement of the talar head. A lateral subtalar dislocation occurs due to an eversion injury and results in lateral displacement of the calcaneus and medial displacement of the talar head. Posterior and anterior subtalar dislocations can also occur, and are the result of a fall from height onto a plantar-flexed or dorsiflexed foot, respectively. These injuries are rare.

3. Early complications include infection and neurovascular injury. An important late complication is osteonecrosis of the talus. It occurs secondary to disruption of the blood supply during the initial injury. Patients may also suffer from persistent instability, post-traumatic arthritis, and osteoporosis.

4. Total talar dislocation is disruption of the subtalar joints (talocalcaneal and talonavicular joint), and the tibiotalar joint [Figures 14 and 15]. It is a serious injury and has a high incidence of subsequent avascular necrosis (AVN) of the talus. It is often an open injury and requires surgical reduction. These injuries are considered an extension of subtalar

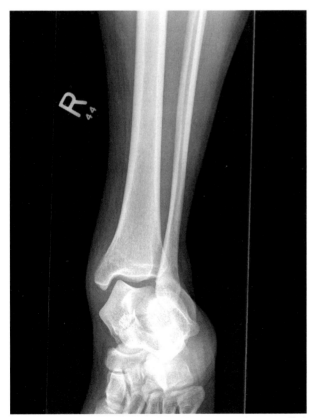

Figure 14. Frontal radiograph demonstrating medial talar subluxation, as well as disruption of the subtalar joint. Although not well appreciated on the plain film, there is an associated fracture of the lateral malleolus (Figure 15).

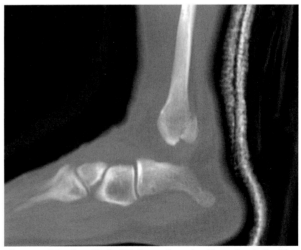

Figure 15. Sagittal CT imaging better depicts the mildly displaced fracture of the lateral malleolus.

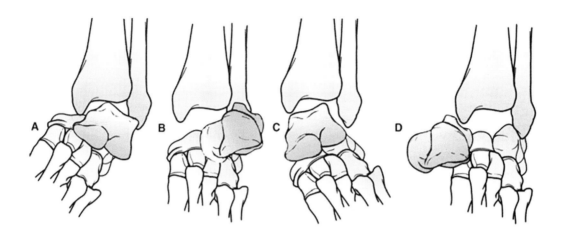

Figure 16. Medial subtalar dislocation (A) is followed by lateral talar subluxation and then eventually total lateral talar dislocation (B). Lateral subtalar dislocation (C) is followed by medial talar subluxation and then eventually total medial talar dislocation (D). *Reprinted with permission from The Journal of Bone and Joint Surgery, Inc. Leitner B. The mechanism of total dislocation of the talus. J Bone Joint Surg 1955; 37A: 93.*

dislocations. For example, a medial subtalar dislocation is followed by lateral talar subluxation and subsequent total lateral talar dislocation (in the setting of continued supination). Lateral subtalar dislocation is followed by medial talar subluxation and subsequent total medial talar dislocation (in the setting of continued pronation) [Figure 16].

Management

A talar dislocation should be reduced as soon as possible. With associated tarsal bone injuries, the reduction can be unstable and difficult due to excessive swelling. However, it should be attempted with the patient splinted appropriately to maintain the reduction. The patient can be consciously sedated if time permits. The knee of the affected extremity is flexed to decrease the tension of the gastrosoleus muscles. Longitudinal traction is applied to initially recreate and exaggerate the deformity to unlock the calcaneus and any debris that may block reduction,

and then the maneuver is performed. For a medial dislocation, the knee is flexed by the assistant, the surgeon applies longitudinal traction to the affected extremity, while simultaneously hyperinverting the foot. The foot is then taken from hyperinversion to eversion. A 'clunk' is felt as the talus falls back into position. The patient can then be placed in a long posterior splint, with or without a U-slab. The opposite maneuver is performed for a lateral dislocation. A CT scan of the talus should then be done to evaluate for any additional fractures, or residual subluxation. If the joint is reduced without associated fractures, the patient is kept non-weight bearing for approximately three weeks, and then ankle range of motion and advancement in weight bearing are begun. If there are associated fractures, these require ORIF.

Total talar dislocations, as in the case above, usually present as open injuries. Initially in the ER any obvious debris in the joint should be removed, and the opening into the joint irrigated. Next, reduction using the above maneuvers, depending on the direction of dislocation, should be performed. The patient is splinted and taken to the operating theater where a more thorough irrigation is performed. The soft tissues are treated carefully and, if appropriate, ORIF can be performed if there is minimal swelling and adequate soft tissue coverage. Often the talus is difficult to reduce in the ER, and a broad incision for an open reduction is done in the operating theater.

Key points

♦ Total talar dislocation is dislocation of the articulations of the talus at the talocalcaneal, talonavicular, and tibiotalar joints.

♦ Medial subtalar dislocation is the most common form, occurring in approximately 85% of cases.

♦ There are often associated fractures involving the tarsal bones, which are better appreciated on a CT study.

♦ Reduction is performed by first exaggerating and re-creating the injury, and then by opposing the direction of injury.

References

1. Karasick D. Fractures and dislocations of the foot. *Semin Roentgenol* 1994; 29(2): 152-75.

2. Leitner B. The mechanism of total dislocation of the talus. *J Bone Joint Surg* 1955; 37A: 93.

3. Palomo-Traver JM, Cruz-Renovell E, *et al.* Open talar dislocation: case report and review of literature. *J Ort Trau* 1997; 11: 45-9.

4. Bohay DR, Manoli A 2nd. Subtalar joint dislocations. *Foot Ankle Int* 1995; 16(12): 803-8.

5. Delee J. Fractures and dislocation of the foot. In: *Surgery of the Foot and Ankle*, 6th ed. Coughlin MJ, Mann RA, Eds. St. Louis, MO: Mosby Inc., 1993: 1465-597.

6. Milenkovic S, Radenkovic M, Mitkovic M. Open subtalar dislocation treated by distractional external fixation. *J Orthop Trauma* 2004; 18(9): 638-40.

7. Detenbeck LC, Kelly PC. Total talar dislocation. *J Bone Joint Surg* 1969; 51(A): 283-8.

Case 4

Clinical presentation

A 23-year-old construction worker falls off the scaffolding. He recalls his fall being broken by his left foot. He presents to the ER for further evaluation. On his workup so far, he has no head trauma, and no spinal injuries. He is only complaining of left foot pain. The images below are obtained.

Physical examination

The patient's left foot is swollen, especially over the hindfoot. The skin is intact. He is very tender to range of motion and splints when you attempt to move the ankle. He is not tender over the medial and lateral malleoli, but appears to be tender over the talus. Distally, he has palpable dorsalis pedis and posterior tibial pulses, and there are no sensory deficits.

Review the images below [Figures 17 and 18]. Describe your findings.

Questions

1. What is the diagnosis?

2. What is the mechanism of injury?

3. How are these injuries classified?

4. What additional study will aid in the management?

5. What muscles/ligaments attach to the talus?

6. Describe the vascular supply of the talus.

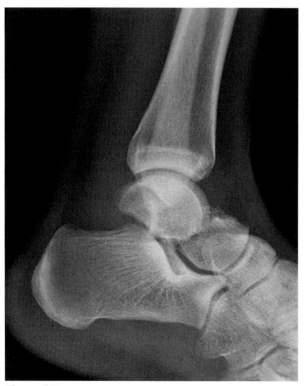

Figure 17.

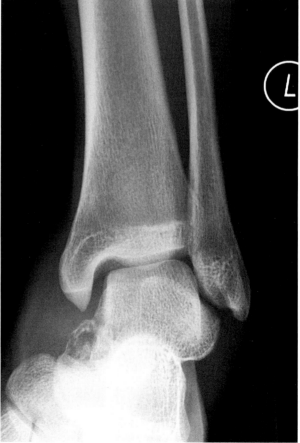

Figure 18.

Radiology findings

On the lateral radiograph, there is a displaced fracture of the talar neck with associated subtalar dislocation. On the frontal radiograph, the ankle joint is intact and no other fractures are present.

Answers

1. Talar neck fracture with subtalar dislocation (Type II).

2. Fractures of the talar neck are typically the result of high-energy trauma such as a motor vehicle accident. They also occur after a fall from height. The injury happens during hyper-dorsiflexion of the talus as it hits the distal tibia. The traditional name of these fractures is 'aviator's astragalus', or the 'rudder bar fracture' referring to the mechanism of the deceleration and direct impact of the foot on the rudder bar in pilots in old-fashioned light airplane crashes.

3. Talar neck fractures have been classified into four types by the Hawkins classification system:
   i) Type I: non-displaced fracture of the talar neck with an intact subtalar joint;
   ii) Type II: fracture associated with either subtalar subluxation or dislocation;
   iii) Type III: fracture associated with subtalar and ankle dislocation;
   iv) Type IV: fracture associated with subtalar joint subluxation and talonavicular joint dislocation.

4. Conservative management of a talar neck fracture is only appropriate with a non-displaced injury. Plain radiographs often times do not accurately show the amount of displacement so a CT scan of the affected extremity should be obtained to better evaluate the fracture fragments and the articular surface.

5. No muscles or tendons have their origins or insertions on the talus.

6. The talus receives its blood supply from branches of the posterior tibial and dorsalis pedis arteries, which pass retrograde from the neck to the body. Therefore, a fracture of the talar neck with displacement is at risk for AVN, making reduction of the joint urgent. Aside from the capsular vessels, the dorsalis pedis artery supplies a branch to the sinus tarsi, and the posterior tibial artery gives rise to the artery of the tarsal canal and the deltoid artery.

Management

If an injury is truly a Type I injury, and non-displaced, it can be treated in a short leg cast, with the patient kept non-weight bearing for 6-8 weeks. The patient is allowed to bear weight as their symptoms improve and X-rays show signs of healing.

For displaced injuries, the fracture should be reduced as soon as possible to prevent AVN. If the joint is adequately reduced in the ER, a follow-up CT scan should be obtained to evaluate for any displacement. If there is displacement, then the patient should be admitted and taken to the operating theater for an ORIF of the talus. If there is no displacement, then the patient can be treated as a Type I injury. If the initial talar injury presents as an open injury, or is irreducible in the ER, the patient should be taken to the operating theater for intervention. The displaced fragment is fixed with lag screws. Postoperatively the patient is also placed in a cast and kept non-weight bearing for approximately 6-8 weeks. The fracture is monitored for signs of AVN.

Key points

- Talar neck/body fractures are severe injuries. Any displaced fractures should be reduced as soon as possible.
- The vascular supply to the talus is fragile, and AVN of the body fragment is common after talar neck fractures.
- In order to treat a fracture conservatively, there should be no displacement. A CT scan can be obtained to evaluate this.
- Patients with talar neck/body fractures should be evaluated for other associated foot injuries. Close attention should be paid to the ankle and talonavicular joints.

References

1.   Vallier HA, Nork SE, Barei DP, Benirschke SK, Sangeorzan BJ. Talar neck fractures: results and outcomes. *J Bone Joint Surg [Am]* 2004; 86: 1616-24.

2.   Lawrence SJ, Singhal M. Open hindfoot injuries. *J Am Acad Orthop Surg* 2007; 15: 367-76.

3.   Chao, Wen, Mizel, Mark S. What's new in foot and ankle surgery? *J Bone Joint Surg [Am]* 2006; 88: 909-22.

4.   Hawkins LG. Fractures of the neck of the talus. *J Bone Joint Surg* 1970; 52: 991-1002

5.   Penny JN, Davis LA. Fractures and fracture: dislocations of the neck of the talus. *J Trauma* 1980; 20: 1029-37.

6.   Lorentzen JE, Christensen SB, Krogsoe O, Sneppen O. Fractures of the neck of the talus. *Acta Orthop Scand* 1977; 48: 115-20.

Case 5

Clinical presentation

A 27-year-old male rugby player presents to the ER with persistent ankle tenderness. He is having trouble practicing and recalls an inversion injury of the ankle that occurred approximately one week prior to presentation. He has been having trouble with his ankle since then. He has rested his ankle, iced it, and elevated it, but has found no relief.

Physical examination

There is swelling over the posterior ankle, but the skin is intact. The patient is tender when the posterior aspect of his ankle is palpated. He has pain with ankle and subtalar range of motion, and with flexion of the great toe. There are no neurovascular deficits.

Review the image below [Figure 19]. Describe your findings.

Questions

1. What is the diagnosis?

2. What is the mechanism of injury?

3. Describe the normal anatomy of the anatomic area injured.

4. What important complication may occur?

5. Why does the patient have pain with great toe plantarflexion?

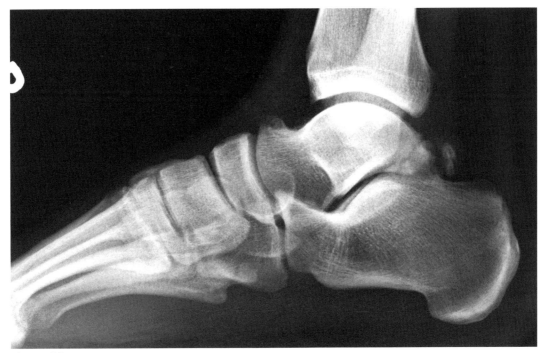

Figure 19.

Radiology findings

There is a displaced fracture of the lateral tubercle of the posterior process of the talus. There are no other fractures. A CT examination further confirms this finding [Figures 20 and 21].

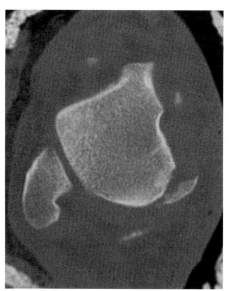

Figure 20. Axial CT image confirms an irregular, displaced fracture of the posterior process of the talus.

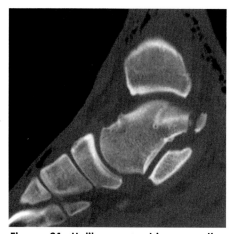

Figure 21. Unlike an os trigonum, the fractured posterior process is irregular and not well corticated, as seen on the sagittal CT image.

Answers

1. Fracture of the posterior process of the talus, involving the lateral tubercle (Shepherd's fracture) [Figure 22].

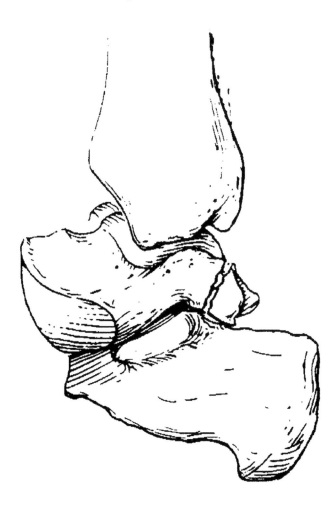

Figure 22. A lateral view of the ankle shows the typical appearance of a fracture of the lateral tubercle of the posterior talar process, also known as a Shepherd's fracture. *Reprinted with permission from the Radiological Society of North America. Hunter T, Peltier L, Lund P, et al. Radiologic history exhibit. Musculoskeletal eponyms: who are those guys? Radiographics 2000; 20(3): 819-36.*

2. Talar process fractures are usually the result of low-energy injuries (such as sporting injuries). Fractures of the lateral and medial tubercles of

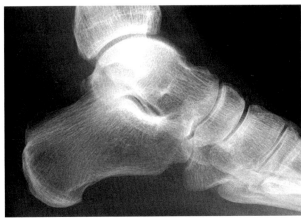

Figure 23. Lateral radiograph of the foot demonstrates the presence of an os trigonum, which can be mistaken for a fracture of the posterior process of the talus. It appears well corticated and smooth.

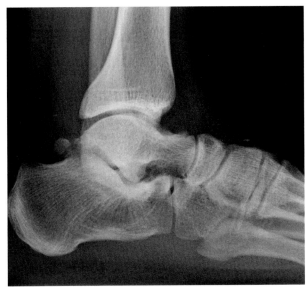

Figure 24. Another lateral radiograph demonstrates an os trigonum.

the posterior process are often involved, and occur due to inversion and eversion mechanisms, respectively. Direct compression injuries can also result in this fracture pattern.

3. The posterior process of the talus is made up of two tubercles: medial and lateral. These tubercles are separated by a groove which contains the flexor hallucis longus tendon. The lateral tubercle is the larger tubercle and projects more posteriorly. It contains the attachment for the posterior talofibular ligament. The medial tubercle contains the attachment for the posterior third of the deltoid ligament. During an inversion injury, the posterior talofibular ligament can cause an avulsion of the lateral tubercle. In an eversion injury, the deltoid ligament can cause an avulsion of the medial tubercle. An important distinction to make is a fracture of the lateral tubercle versus an os trigonum, a normal feature just posterior to the lateral tubercle [Figures 23 and 24]. Unlike an acute fracture, the edges of an os trigonum are well corticated and smooth. A high index of suspicion, and often a CT scan, are necessary to make the diagnosis.

4. Non-union of fracture fragments at the lateral tubercle of the posterior talar process is important to recognize, because it may require surgical involvement including excision of the non-united fragment. Patients often complain of pain with plantarflexion, and physical activity. On physical examination, they have restricted ankle and subtalar joint motion. Another important complication to be aware of due to non-union is partial rupture or tenosynovitis of the flexor hallucis longus tendon.

5. Pain occurs with great toe flexion as the flexor hallucis longus runs over the fracture site.

Management

Diagnosing these injuries is difficult. Often, patients attribute their pain to a very bad ankle sprain, as in this case, and present only after no relief is found with rest, ice, and elevation. A CT scan can help to differentiate an os trigonum from a displaced versus minimally displaced fracture of the posterior process of the talus. For minimally displaced fractures, the patient can be placed in a short leg cast, and kept non-weight bearing for 4-6 weeks. For displaced fractures with a large avulsed fragment, ORIF with screw placement may be required. However, if the fragment is very small then excision of the fragment is performed.

Key points

- Fractures of the posterior talus can involve either the medial or lateral tubercle.
- They must be distinguished from an os trigonum, which arises posterior to the lateral tubercle.
- Minimally displaced fractures can be treated in a cast.
- A CT scan should be obtained to evaluate the amount of displacement of the involved fragment.

References

1. Hunter TB, Peltier LF, Lund PJ. Radiologic history exhibit. Musculoskeletal eponyms: who are those guys? *Radiographics* 2000; 20(3): 819-36.

2. Higgins TF, Baumgaertner MR. Diagnosis and treatment of fractures of the talus: a comprehensive review of the literature. *Foot Ankle Int* 1999; 20(9): 595-605.

3. Hawkins LG. Fracture of the lateral process of the talus. *J Bone Joint Surg [Am]* 1965; 47: 1170-5.

Case 6

Clinical presentation

A 22-year-old girl presents to the ER after landing on her feet from a jump out of her third story window. She was trying to jump over to the tree outside her dorm room, and missed. She reports twisting her left ankle when she fell, and now has persistent pain in her left foot. The ER evaluation is negative for any associated spinal injuries.

Physical examination

There is significant swelling and bruising over the dorsum of the foot. The skin is intact. The patient has pain on palpation most significantly between the first and second metatarsals. A posterior tibial pulse is palpable. The dorsalis pedis pulse is not palpable through the swelling, but can be detected with Doppler with good biphasic flow.

Review the images below [Figures 25 and 26]. Describe your findings.

Questions

1. What is the diagnosis?

2. What is the mechanism of injury?

3. How is this injury classified?

4. Describe the normal Lisfranc joint. What bones does it include? How does it normally appear on radiographs?

5. What complications can arise from this type of injury?

6. On radiographs, what signs would you look for that may suggest a Lisfranc injury?

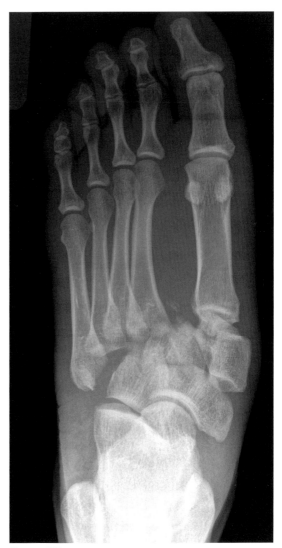

Figure 25.

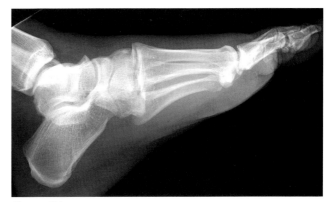

Figure 26.

Radiology findings

There is an 11mm diastasis (widening) between the bases of the first and second metatarsals. There is subsequent lateral migration of the second through fifth metatarsals. There is also lateral migration of the first metatarsal. There is malalignment of the medial margin of the second metatarsal base and the medial edge of the middle (second) cuneiform. There are multiple bony fragments projected around the Lisfranc joint including one just proximal to the fifth metatarsal and another adjacent to the cuboid. These indicate a positive flake sign (multiple avulsed bone fragments centered around the Lisfranc joint), suggesting severe ligamentous injury to the Lisfranc ligament and joint disruption. There are smaller bony fragments which seem to originate from the distal aspects of the cuneiforms. A fracture of the base of the second metatarsal is not definitely appreciated. On the lateral view, there is dorsal displacement of the metatarsals, indicating ligamentous compromise.

Answers

1. Lisfranc fracture-dislocation [Figure 27].

2. This injury is caused by forced plantar flexion of the foot and twisting on landing from a fall. These injuries can occur via a direct force (for example, a heavy object falling on the dorsum of the foot) or indirectly via violent forced plantar flexion or twisting of the forefoot, as in this case. Forced plantar flexion injuries often are accompanied with fractures of the metatarsals, whereas twisting injuries (aggressive abduction) are usually accompanied by ligamentous injury and fractures of the cuboid and the base of the second metatarsal.

3. In the Quenu and Kuss system, these injuries are classified into three groups:
    i) Type A injuries are homolateral injuries, with displacement of all five metatarsals in the same direction. Since the second metatarsal is keyed into the metatarsotarsal joint, in order for this injury pattern to occur there is usually a fracture at the base of the second metatarsal;

    ii) Type B injuries are isolated injuries, with displacement of one or two metatarsals away from the others;
    iii) Type C injuries are divergent injuries, with displacement of the metatarsals in both the sagittal and coronal planes. The second to fifth metatarsals are displaced laterally and the first metatarsal is displaced medially or

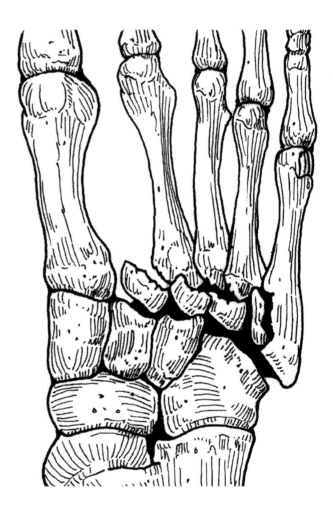

Figure 27. Schematic drawing of a Lisfranc fracture-dislocation. *Reprinted with permission from the Radiological Society of North America. Hunter T, Peltier L, Lund P, et al. Musculoskeletal eponyms: who are those guys? Radiographics 2000; 20(3): 819-36.*

dorsally. Again, since the second metatarsal is depressed compared with metatarsals three to five, in order for this injury pattern to occur there is usually a fracture through the base of the second metatarsal.

The Myerson classification system describes the direction of injury and aids in identifying which elements of the injury need to be repaired. In total incongruity, the direction of injury can be either lateral, or dorsal/plantar. Unlike in partial incongruity where there is often medial displacement of the first metatarsal compared to the rest of the toes, in total incongruity the first metatarsal and the remaining toes all dislocate in the same direction. In partial incongruity there is either medial or lateral dislocation of the second metatarsal in relation to the medial cuneiform. In a divergent pattern there is lateral displacement of the second metatarsal in relation to the medial cuneiform, with associated medial displacement of the first metatarsal.

4. The Lisfranc joint is the base of the second metatarsal which fits into a socket formed by the first, second and third cuneiforms. Reduction and stability of this joint is the key to understanding and managing the Lisfranc injury. The Lisfranc ligament is the most important in ensuring stability. It attaches the medial cuneiform to the base of the second metatarsal. On AP radiographs, the medial border of the second metatarsal should align with the medial border of the middle cuneiform. The medial border of the fourth metatarsal should align with the medial border of the cuboid (oblique view). Dorsal displacement of the metatarsals on a lateral radiograph indicates ligamentous compromise.

5. Patients may suffer from compartment syndrome due to swelling. This should always be considered although decompression of foot compartments is controversial. The dorsalis pedis artery runs between the first and second metatarsals, and can be lacerated in this injury.

Other complications include post-traumatic arthritis, reflex sympathetic dystrophy, complex mediated regional pain syndrome and infection after wound breakdown.

6. Lisfranc injuries can also be subtle, and up to 20% are missed on initial radiographs. Dislocation of the tarsometatarsal joint is indicated by: loss of alignment between the lateral margin of the first metatarsal and the lateral edge of the medial cuneiform; loss of alignment between the medial margin of the second metatarsal and the medial edge of the middle cuneiform; loss of alignment between the medial border of the fourth metatarsal and the medial border of the cuboid (oblique view); the presence of small bone fragments around the Lisfranc joint (flake sign); and dorsal displacement of the metatarsals relative to the tarsals (lateral view). CT images are useful to further delineate fractures and intra-articular extension.

Management

In this case, the injury involves all five metatarsals, with significant dorsolateral displacement of the second through fifth metatarsals. The reduction maneuver is therefore performed with a plantar-medial force, with the midfoot stabilized by screws angled from medial to lateral to hold the second metatarsal to the medial cuneiform and subsequent screws passed to stabilize all elements of the fracture. This can be accomplished open or closed; if closed, anatomic reduction is essential and screws can then be placed percutaneously. Many surgeons prefer to open the area of the base of the second metatarsal to confirm that the reduction of this key structure is anatomic.

Lisfranc injuries are frequently not as obvious as in this case. When patients complain of foot pain and have an initial presentation of 'ankle sprain' it is difficult to asses for Lisfranc injuries, and these can be missed. Further assessment for persisting suspicion of this injury may include weight bearing views of the foot, CT scans or plain film radiographs under anesthesia to assess suspected midfoot instability.

Key points

♦ The joint at the base of the second metatarsal is the critical aspect of the Lisfranc injury as it keys into a socket against the middle cuneiform. Anatomic reduction of this is essential. If there is a fracture through the base of the second metatarsal in line with the remaining metatarsals, then on reduction the shaft of the second metatarsal needs to be appropriately aligned with the depressed proximal portion that has remained attached to the medial cuneiform in order to re-establish normal anatomy and function.

♦ The Lisfranc ligament is one of the most important ligaments at the base of the foot. It attaches from the medial cuneiform to the base of the second metatarsal.

♦ The third through fifth metatarsals often reduce as the second metatarsal is appropriately aligned.

♦ Lisfranc injuries can be difficult to diagnose, and one should be wary of an ankle sprain injury with persistent pain. These patients should be re-evaluated with weight bearing views of their injured foot.

References

1. Heckman JD. Fractures and dislocations of the foot. In: *Rockwood and Green's Fractures in Adults*, Vol 2, 3rd ed. Rockwood CA, Green DP, Bucholz RW, Eds. Philadelphia, PA: Lippincott, 1991: 2140-51.

2. Bucholz RW, Heckman JD, Court-Brown C, *et al*, Eds. *Rockwood and Green's Fractures in Adults*, 6th ed. Philadelphia, PA: Lippincott Williams & Wilkins, 2006.

3. Myerson MS, Fisher RT, Burgess AR, *et al*. Fracture-dislocations of the tarsometatarsal joints: end results correlated with pathology and treatment. *Foot Ankle* 1986; 6: 225-42.

4. Hardcastle PH, Reschauer R, Kitscha-Lissberg E, *et al*. Injuries to the tarsometatarsal joint: incidence, classification and treatment. *J Bone Joint Surg [Br]* 1982; 64B: 349.

5. Wiley JJ. The mechanism of tarso-metatarsal joint injuries. *J Bone Joint Surg [Br]* 1971; 53: 474-82.

6. Kraeger DR. Foot injuries. In: *Handbook of Sports Medicine: a Symptom-oriented Approach*. Lillegard WA, Rucker KS, Eds. Boston, MA: Andover Medical, 1993: 159-71.

7. Hunter T, Peltier L, Lund P. Musculoskeletal eponyms: who are those guys? *Radiographics* 2000; 20(3): 819-36.

Case 7

Clinical presentation

A 25-year-old healthy male twisted his right foot/ankle while playing basketball. He describes an inversion type injury, with subsequent swelling and pain on the lateral border of the foot. He is able to weight bear but with pain.

Physical examination

There is pain and swelling over the lateral aspect of the right foot, mostly over the proximal fifth metatarsal. The skin is intact. There is tenderness to palpation over the fifth metatarsal. His ankle exam is benign.

Review the image below [Figure 28]. Describe your findings.

Questions

1. What is the diagnosis?

2. How would you distinguish a Jones fracture from a 'pseudo-Jones fracture' on plain films?

3. What would be your initial management in the ER?

4. What is the main complication with these fractures?

5. What are the differential diagnoses?

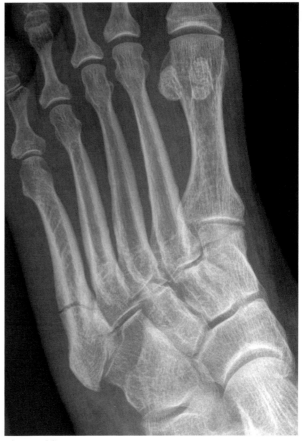

Figure 28.

Radiology findings

There is a linear fracture of the fifth metatarsal bone at the metaphyseal-diaphyseal junction. Of note, the fracture line is distal to the tuberosity of the fifth metatarsal. The fracture margins are sharp and there is no intramedullary sclerosis. These findings are compatible with an acute Jones fracture.

Answers

1. Jones fracture.

2. A pseudo-Jones fracture is an avulsion fracture of the base of the fifth metatarsal by the peroneus brevis tendon [Figure 29]. It involves the cancellous tuberosity, differentiating it from a true Jones fracture.

3. Initially in the ER, the patient should be put into a short leg cast, and told to non-weight bear on the right lower extremity.

4. Non-union is a frequent concern with these fractures, and they often go on to require operative fixation.

5. Other differential diagnoses include a normal apophysis, an os peroneum and a stress fracture.

Management

Management is with a short leg cast versus screw fixation. The fifth metatarsal is divided into three zones [Figure 30]. Zone 1 injuries are often avulsion injuries, and are treated with a hard sole shoe. Zone 3 injuries (stress fractures) are rare, but they have a tendency

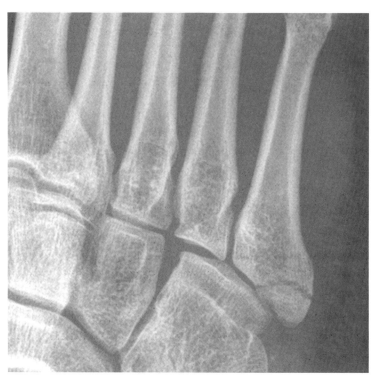

Figure 29. There is a non-displaced fracture at the base of the fifth metatarsal, at the metaphysis and proximal to the metatarsocuboid joint. There is no angulation or intra-articular extension of the fracture line. These findings are consistent with a pseudo-Jones fracture.

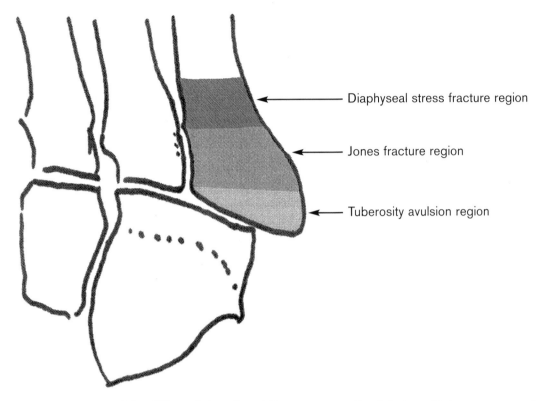

Diaphyseal stress fracture region

Jones fracture region

Tuberosity avulsion region

Figure 30. Three zones of the fifth metatarsal and the corresponding injuries which may occur. *Reprinted with permission from the Radiological Society of North America. Stevens M, El-Khoury G, Kathol M, et al. Imaging features of avulsion injuries. Radiographics 1999; 19: 655-72.*

for non-union and often require operative fixation. Jones fractures are in Zone 2. A fracture in Zone 2 should be treated as a Jones fracture.

Key points

- A Jones fracture is a fracture of the base of the fifth metatarsal at the metaphyseal-diaphyseal junction.

- It should be differentiated from a pseudo-Jones fracture, which is an avulsion fracture of the base of the fifth metatarsal and most commonly involves non-operative management.

- Jones fractures may initially be managed with a short leg cast, but may require screw fixation if they fail to heal.

References

1. Dameron TB. Fractures of the proximal fifth metatarsal: selecting the best treatment option. *J Am Acad Ortho Surg* 1995; 3: 110-4.

2. Koval KJ, Zuckerman JD. *Handbook of Fractures*, 3rd ed. Philadelphia, PA: Lippincott Williams & Wilkins, 2006.

Case 8

Clinical presentation

A 20-year-old ballerina injures her right foot after a jump. She notes pain on the lateral aspect of her right foot, and presents to the ER for further evaluation.

Physical examination

There is swelling over the lateral aspect of the right foot. The skin is intact, and there is no bruising or gross deformity. There is tenderness to palpation over the right metatarsal. The patient has pain with range of motion of her small toe. There are no associated neurovascular injuries.

Review the image below [Figure 31]. Describe your findings.

Questions

1. What is the diagnosis?

2. What is the mechanism of injury?

3. What function does the forefoot serve?

4. How are fifth metatarsal injuries classified?

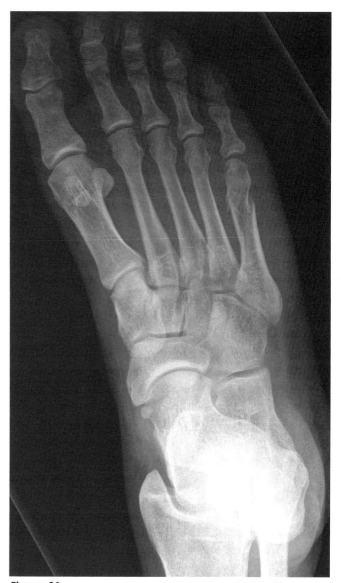

Figure 31.

Radiology findings

There is a spiral fracture involving the distal shaft of the fifth metatarsal. A maximal amount of displacement is seen to 3mm.

Answers

1. Metatarsal shaft fracture.

2. Fractures of the metatarsal shaft most often occur after a direct blow (due to a heavy object falling on the foot), or due to a twisting mechanism (termed Dancer's fracture, as in the case above).

3. The forefoot serves as a load bearing and distributing surface in gait. The metatarsals are also mobile in the sagittal plane. This allows people to walk relatively comfortably on uneven ground without breaking any of the forefoot bones, as the foot is able to accommodate the surface.

4. Fifth metatarsal injuries are divided into proximal base injuries, and distal spiral, or Dancer's fracture injuries. Proximal base injuries are further divided into three zones, and treatment varies based on the zone of fracture (for further discussion, see the case on Jones fracture). Dancer's fractures make up the majority of distal injuries. These fractures are spiral or oblique, and the fracture pattern is that as seen above, with the fracture progressing from lateral to medial, and distal to proximal.

Management

Dancer's fractures are treated symptomatically. Patients are initially told to rest, and ice and elevate the affected leg. They are placed in supportive immobilization based on their degree of discomfort, which can range from a short leg cast or splint to a stiff soled shoe. Patients may need support to walk but can weight bear as tolerated. Progressive healing over a few weeks with minimal or no long-term disability would be expected.

Key points

- Fifth metatarsal fractures are usually a result of a twisting injury or a direct blow.
- They are divided into proximal and distal fractures.
- The fracture pattern of distal fractures is usually oblique or spiral moving from lateral to medial, and distal to proximal.
- Treatment of these fractures is symptomatic.

References

1. Quill GE. Fractures of the proximal fifth metatarsal. *Orthop Clin North Am* 1995; 26(2): 353-61.

2. Lawrence SJ, Botte MJ. Jones' fractures and related fractures of the proximal fifth metatarsal. *Foot Ankle* 1993; 14(6): 358-65.

3. Wiener BD, Linder JF, Giattini JF. Treatment of fractures of the fifth metatarsal: a prospective study. *Foot Ankle Int* 1997; 18: 267.

4. Holubec KD, Karlin JM, Scurran BL. Retrospective study of fifth metatarsal fractures. *J Am Podiatr Med Assoc* 1993; 83: 215.

Case 9

Clinical presentation

A 22-year-old basketball player presents after landing hard on his right foot after shooting a hoop, and twisting his ankle as he lands. He complains of severe pain that started immediately, and is unable to bear weight on his right foot after having limped off the court with the help of his trainer.

Physical examination

The right foot is swollen dorsolaterally. The skin is intact. There is pain with palpation, and ecchymosis. There are no neurovascular deficits.

Review the image below [Figure 32]. Describe your findings.

Questions

1. What is the likely diagnosis?

2. What is the mechanism of injury?

3. What complications may arise?

4. What is cuboid syndrome?

5. Describe the anatomy of the midfoot.

6. Describe three functions of the cuboid.

7. If the cuboid dislocates, what is the direction of dislocation?

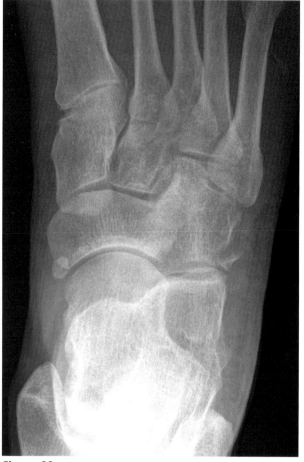

Figure 32.

Radiology findings

There is a fracture of the cuboid partially involving the calcaneocuboid joint space orientated in the sagittal plane. There is less than 2mm displacement and no evidence for cuboid subluxation or loss of bony length.

Answers

1. Cuboid fracture.

2. Injuries to the cuboid can result from both low-energy (simple ankle twisting) and high-energy (motor vehicle accident, direct blow) mechanisms. There is usually forced plantar flexion and abduction. An isolated injury to the cuboid is uncommon. It is often associated with talonavicular joint injuries, Lisfranc injuries, and other midfoot structures. It may represent instability of the whole lateral column of the midfoot.

3. In addition to general fracture complications, cuboid fractures may result in instability and post-traumatic arthritis. Patients may also suffer from loss of lateral column length, which results in pain and an altered gait.

4. Cuboid syndrome is a poorly understood phenomenon, resulting in misdiagnosis and mistreatment. It is defined as a subluxation or disruption of the calcaneocuboid portion of the midtarsal joint, resulting in irritation of the surrounding joint capsule, ligaments and peroneus longus tendon. Various etiologies have been proposed, the most common school of thought being that this syndrome results from plantar flexion and inversion ankle sprains. Patients present with pain over the cuboid that has gradually worsened over time after a previous minor ankle sprain. Radiographs are usually negative. Patients generally respond well to conservative management often with placement of a supportive pad under the medial portion of the cuboid.

5. The cuboid is located in the midfoot. The midfoot is distal to Chopart's joint (talonavicular and calcaneocuboid joints) and proximal to the Lisfranc joint (tarsometatarsal joint). Distally, the cuboid articulates with the fourth and fifth metatarsals, and proximally it articulates with the anterior calcaneus. The metatarsocuboid articulation is more important to overall foot function than the calcaneocuboid articulation. The five bones in the midfoot are the navicular, cuboid, medial cuneiform, middle cuneiform and lateral cuneiform. There is very little motion in the midfoot. The midfoot is more rigid, and serves to help unite the more mobile forefoot and hindfoot. Therefore, distortions in the midfoot can also disrupt the mechanics of the forefoot and hindfoot. The cuboid is part of the lateral support column of the foot.

6. The three functions of the cuboid are:
   i) structural support for the lateral column of the foot;
   ii) articulation with the fourth and fifth metatarsals;
   iii) calcaneocuboid joint motion.

7. The direction of dislocation of the cuboid is plantar and medial.

Management

For isolated cuboid fractures, without loss of length and no instability, treatment is non-operative. The patient should be placed in a cast and kept non-weight bearing for 4-6 weeks. For small avulsion injuries, with no loss of length or instability (as in the case above), the patient is also treated non-operatively. The patient should be provided with a walking boot, and allowed to be weight bearing as tolerated.

In general for cuboid fractures, non-operative treatment is considered if there is less than 2mm displacement at the articular surface of the cuboid, no subluxation, and no loss of length. Patients are treated in a cast for 4-6 weeks. They are kept non-weight bearing if the injury is a fracture, and weight bearing as tolerated in an air cast boot if the injury is an avulsion. X-rays are repeated at 7-10 days to confirm maintenance of position. Operative intervention is considered if there is significant fracture displacement or dislocation of the calcaneocuboid joint. A variety of fixation methods ranging from Kirschner wire to screw or mini plate fixation can be implemented. Appropriate postoperative cast protection will be required.

Key points

- In treating the midfoot, stability is an important major aim to keep the forefoot and hindfoot well aligned.
- The direction of dislocation of the cuboid is always plantar and medial.
- In general if there is minimal displacement, there is a low risk of malalignment of the forefoot and hindfoot, and these fractures can be treated conservatively. If there is significant displacement, operative fixation is considered.

References

1. Miller C, Winter W, Bucknell A, *et al.* Injuries to the midtarsal joint and lesser tarsal bones. *J Am Acad Orthop Surg* 1998; 6: 249-58.
2. Blakeslee TJ, Morris JL. Cuboid syndrome and the significance of midtarsal joint stability. *Journal of the American Podiatry Medical Association* 1987; 77(12): 638-42.
3. Newell SG, Woodle A. Cuboid syndrome. *Physician and Sports Medicine* 1981; 9: 71-6.
4. Bucholz RW, Heckman JD, Court-Brown CM, *et al,* Eds. *Rockwood and Green's Fractures in Adults*, 6th ed. Philadelphia, PA: Lippincott Williams & Wilkins, 2006.

Case 10

Clinical presentation

A 22-year-old man was mowing the lawn at a golf course. His left leg became briefly caught under the mower. He was able to pull out his leg from underneath; however, he was injured by the blade as he withdrew his foot. He is brought to the ER by his colleagues.

Physical examination

The skin over the medial foot is open, and bone is visible through the opening. There are palpable dorsalis pedis and posterior tibial pulses. The patient has decreased sensation over the medial aspect of his foot as well as on the dorsomedial aspect of his foot.

Despite his discomfort, he is able to dorsiflex, plantarflex, and evert his foot. The most significant finding is difficulty with inversion.

Review the images below [Figures 33 and 34]. Describe your findings.

Questions

1. What is the diagnosis?

2. What is the mechanism of injury?

3. How are these injuries classified?

4. Describe the anatomy of the navicular bone.

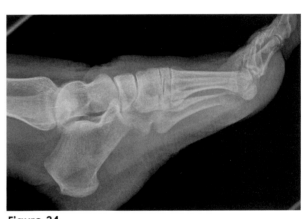

Figure 34.

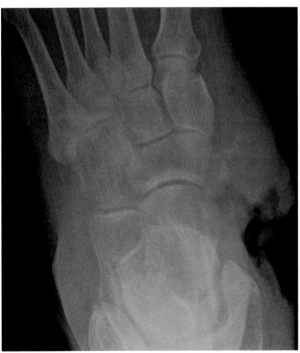

Figure 33.

Radiology findings

There is irregularity of the soft tissue over the medial aspect of the foot. There is cortical disruption and posterior displacement of the medial navicular bone, and cortical disruption at the talonavicular joint.

Answers

1. Open navicular tuberosity fracture.

2. Navicular tuberosity fractures are as a result of a combination of traction and eversion of the foot. These forces cause bony avulsion as the deltoid ligament and posterior tibial tendon are stretched. In this case, the patient probably sustained the fracture during the fall and tug under the lawn mower, and the open injury just proximal is likely due to the lawnmower blade after the fracture occurred.

3. There are three basic types of navicular fractures. Descriptive terms are used to describe these types. They include avulsion fractures (the most common), tuberosity fractures, and body fractures. The navicular body fractures are further sub-classified into three types:
   i) Type I body fractures split the navicular bone in the lateral plane into a dorsal and plantar segment;
   ii) Type II body fractures split the navicular bone in the AP plane into a medial and lateral segment;
   iii) Type III body fractures involve comminution of a fracture segment in the AP plane, with significant displacement of both medial and lateral segments.

4. The navicular bone is a key support of the medial arch of the foot. In terms of size, the bone is wider dorsally and medially compared with its size plantar and laterally. Its proximal surface articulates with the talus, and its distal surface articulates with each of the cuneiforms, which helps to dissipate forces across the foot. The navicular tuberosity is the site of attachment of the posterior tibial tendon. This is usually avulsed during an avulsion type injury.

Management

Isolated injuries of the navicular bone are rare due to its close relationship with the other tarsal bones. Therefore, with any fracture of the navicular bone, additional fractures should be looked for in the foot, especially of the talus and cuneiforms. In this case, there may be a fracture of the talus near the talonavicular joint. If this is a concern, a CT scan can be obtained to better visualize the articular surface.

With an open injury, such as the one above, in the ER the foot should be covered with a sterile dressing, and placed in a posterior splint. The fracture can then be copiously irrigated in the operating theater before fixation of the fragment. In the operating theater, the talonavicular joint should be examined. If it is minimally involved, the talus can be left alone. For an avulsion fracture involving 25% or more of the navicular, this can be reduced using a mini-fragment screw. If less than 25% of the bone is involved, the fragment can simply be excised.

In general, fractures of the navicular bone that cause incongruity of the articular surface should undergo operative fixation. Fractures displaced more than 2mm have been found to be incongruent, and warrant fixation. Reconstruction of the articular surface is considered if >40% of the talonavicular joint can be restored. If less than 40% is amenable to fixation, then the patient often has better function with decreased pain after a talonavicular fusion.

Key points

- Isolated fractures of the navicular are rare.
- The navicular is a keystone of the medial arch of the foot. It articulates with the talus and the three cuneiforms.
- There are three types of navicular fractures: avulsion, tuberosity, and body fractures. Body fractures are further sub-classified into three types.
- Attempt at restoration of the talonavicular articular surface and stability of the medial column of the foot is the goal of operative management.

References

1. Pinney SJ, Sangeorzan BJ. Fractures of the tarsal bones. *Orthop Clin North Am* 2001; 32(1): 21-33.

2. Thordarson DB. Fractures of the midfoot and forefoot. In: *Foot and Ankle Disorders*, 2nd ed. Myerson MS, Leonard ME, Eds. Orlando, FLA: Harcourt, 2000: 1265-85.

3. Coughlin L, Kwok D, Oliver J. Fracture dislocation of the tarsal navicular. A case report. *Am J Sports Med* 1987; 15(6): 614-5.

4. Heckman JD. Fractures and dislocations of the foot. In: *Rockwood and Green's Fractures in Adults*, 4th ed. Rockwood CA, Green DP, Eds. Philadelphia, PA: Lippincott Williams & Wilkins, 1996: 2355-62.

Chapter 9

Pediatric trauma

Case 1

Clinical presentation

A three-year-old boy is playing on the monkey bars when he falls and lands onto his right outstretched hand. He has immediate pain at the elbow and will not use his arm or stop crying. The parents bring him into the ER for evaluation.

Physical examination

On exam, the skin is intact. There is swelling over the elbow, but no ecchymosis. Distally, the patient has palpable radial and ulnar pulses. He can retropulse his thumb, abduct his fingers, and make an OK sign. Sensation is intact in the radial, median, and ulnar nerve distributions.

Review the images below [Figures 1 and 2]. Describe your findings.

Questions

1. What is the diagnosis?

2. What is the mechanism of injury?

3. What is the difference between a flexion and extension type injury?

4. How can you identify the age of the patient based on the ossification centers of the elbow?

5. What classification system is typically used?

6. Why is displacement of the distal fracture fragment important?

7. What is the most common nerve injured in a flexion type injury? What other injuries can occur?

8. Define the anterior humeral line, radiocapitellar line and Baumann angle.

9. When will you not see a posterior fat pad sign on radiographs?

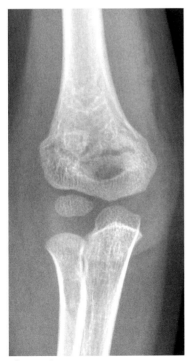

Figure 1.

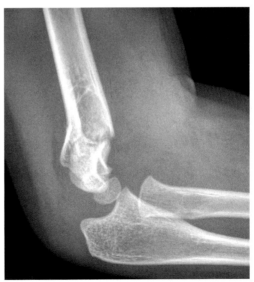

Figure 2.

Radiology findings

There is a transverse supracondylar fracture with dorsal displacement of the distal fracture fragment. The posterior humeral cortex is intact at the fracture line. The distal fragment demonstrates rotation and angulation. Anterior and posterior joint effusions are seen.

Answers

1. Gartland Type II supracondylar fracture.

2. The injury is caused by axial loading onto an extremity with a tight anterior capsule. This allows for the fracture at the anterior humerus to serve as a fulcrum. If the arm is extended and supinated at the time of impact, there is posterior lateral displacement of the distal fragment. If the arm is extended and pronated then there is posterior medial displacement of the distal fragment. In the above case, there is little medial or lateral displacement, likely because the force generated was not large enough to cause complete disruption and displacement.

3. In a flexion type injury, the patient lands with the arm in flexion instead of extension. As a result the distal fragment is displaced anteriorly, as opposed to posteriorly with an extension type injury.

4. The age of a patient can be determined based on the appearance of various structures of the elbow joint (Table 1). These are commonly remembered by the mnemonic 'CRMTOL' with girls given odd numbers 1, 3, 5, 7, 9, 11 and boys given even numbers 2, 4, 6, 8, 10, 12.

In the X-rays above (Figures 1 and 2), the child is a boy, so the mnemonic should be started at even numbers. Only the capitellum is present, therefore the child is between two and four years of age. The importance of this is to confirm that the correct centers of ossification are present. In the incompletely ossified elbow some injuries can be very difficult to assess. In select cases comparison views of the normal side can be helpful.

5. The Gartland system is used to classify supracondylar fractures. This system is based on the radiographic displacement of fracture fragments and is grouped as follows:
   i) Type I: non-displaced fracture without medial or lateral displacement. The anterior humeral line crosses the capitellum;
   ii) Type II: displaced fracture, with an intact posterior cortex;
   iii) Type III: displaced fracture with no contact between the fracture fragments [Figure 3]. There may be a 'T' type fracture, which involves an intracondylar split visualized as a vertical lucent line between the epiphyseal fracture fragments.

Table 1. Determination of a patient's age dependent on the appearance of structures.

Structure	Age at presentation in girls	Age at presentation in boys
Capitellum	1	2
Radial head	3	4
Medial epicondyle	5	6
Trochlea	7	8
Olecranon	9	10
Lateral epicondyle	11	12

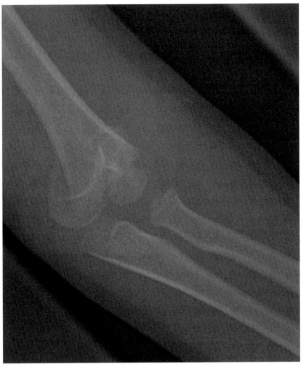 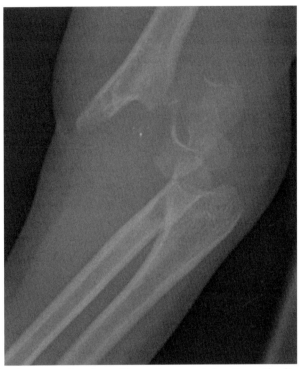

Figure 3. AP and lateral views of a Type III supracondylar humerus fracture. There is complete discontinuity between both anterior and posterior cortices of the proximal humerus and distal fracture fragment. There is also a rotational deformity. The distal fragment is displaced posteromedially.

6. Displacement of the distal humeral fragment is important because it allows the clinician to predict associated injuries. If the distal fragment is displaced medially, the radial nerve is at risk. If the distal fragment is displaced laterally, the median nerve and brachial artery are most at risk.

7. The most common nerve injured in a flexion type injury is the ulnar nerve. Additional injuries include damage to the brachial artery due to a spike of the distal fracture fragment. However, more importantly, is the degree of swelling, especially in badly displaced Type III fractures. Antecubital swelling can compress the brachial artery with a resultant pulseless limb distally. Immediate fracture reduction needs to take place. If there is a delay in getting the patient up to the operating theater, then this reduction should be attempted urgently in the ER.

8. The anterior humeral line is drawn on a lateral radiograph and extends along the anterior aspect of the distal humeral metaphysis through the middle third of the capitellum. Disruption of this line (for example, if it does not pass through the middle third of the capitellum) indicates a fracture. The radiocapitellar line extends from the proximal radius through the capitellum. Disruption of this line indicates dislocation, as it depicts the relationship of the radius to the capitellum. The Baumann angle is determined by a perpendicular line drawn to the humeral shaft and a parallel line drawn through the lateral condyle. It is usually 15°, but should be compared with the opposite side. A posterior fat pad sign is never normal, and can also indicate intra-articular injury. These lines and signs can help identify injuries in a pediatric elbow, which is difficult when all of the bony anatomy is not yet present.

9. A posterior fat pad sign will likely not be visible in a Type III supracondylar fracture, or in an elbow dislocation. This is because the joint capsule is

torn, and therefore there is decompression of the joint and no accumulation of fluid.

Management

Without correction, these fractures can lead to a varus deformity of the elbow. If the vessels are compromised, a Volkmann's contracture of the forearm is a classic late complication.

Management of supracondylar fractures depends on whether the fracture is a flexion or extension type.

Extension-type injuries:

◆ Type I fractures: treated with a long arm cast with the arm flexed at 60-90° at the elbow for approximately three weeks.

◆ Type II fractures: closed manipulation in the operating theater, with percutaneous pinning. If adequate reduction cannot be obtained closed, then the fracture can be opened and then percutaneously pinned. The reduction maneuver for these fractures is to realign the fracture if there is medial or lateral displacement by applying tension in the lateral direction for medial displacement, and medially for lateral displacement. To fix the posterior displacement the elbow is flexed and upward force applied to the olecranon simultaneously. The reduction is checked under C-arm imaging intra-operatively, and reperformed as necessary.

◆ Type III fractures: these fractures are taken to the operating theater for closed reduction and percutaneous pinning. If this is unsuccessful, the fracture is opened to perform the reduction, and then pinned using two to three Kirschner wires. The reduction maneuver is performed as above. If there is persisting vascular compromise, the brachial artery may need to be explored.

Flexion-type injuries:

◆ Type I fractures: long arm cast for approximately three weeks.

◆ Type II fractures: closed reduction with percutaneous pinning. These fractures are often difficult to close reduce and frequently require opening.

◆ Type III: these fractures almost inevitably require opening. Closed reduction can be attempted, but most fractures will require opening. Fixation is again with two to three Kirschner wires across the fracture site.

After reduction, these fractures are casted for three weeks. At three-week follow-up the Kirschner wires are removed, the cast is removed if there is adequate healing, and patients are allowed to resume activity as tolerated. Contact sports should be avoided for at least an additional month.

Key points

◆ Supracondylar fractures are most commonly seen in children between the ages of five and seven years.

◆ They are divided into extension-type (more common) and flexion-type injuries and are classified by the Gartland system.

◆ Most are treated with closed reduction and percutaneous pinning using Kirschner wires.

◆ Radiographically, the anterior humeral line, radiocapitellar line, Baumann's angle, and posterior fat pad sign all help to identify fractures in a developing elbow.

References

1. Gartland JJ. Management of supracondylar fractures of the humerus in children. *Surg Gynecol Obstet* 1959; 109: 145-54.

2. Wilkins KE. Fractures and dislocations of the elbow region. In: *Fractures in Children*. Vol III, 3rd ed. Rockwood CA, Wilkins KE, King RE, Eds. Philadelphia, PA: JB Lippincott; 1984: 540-1.

Case 2

Clinical presentation

A 17-year-old boy, left hand dominant, presents to the ER after falling off his bike and landing onto his left elbow. He felt immediate pain afterwards, and swelling. His mother brings him in for further evaluation.

Physical examination

The left elbow is swollen. Surprisingly, there is no bruising, and the skin is intact. Distally, he can retropulse his thumb, make an OK sign, and spread apart his fingers. He has palpable radial and ulnar pulses. His sensation is intact in radial, median, and ulnar nerve distributions.

Review the images below [Figures 4 and 5]. Describe your findings.

Questions

1. What is the diagnosis?

2. What is the mechanism of injury?

3. What type of injury is this often confused with?

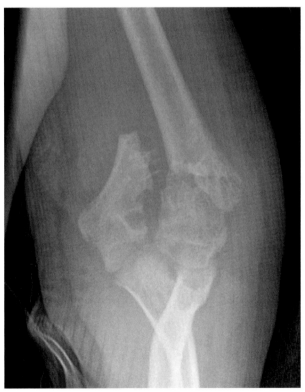

Figure 4.

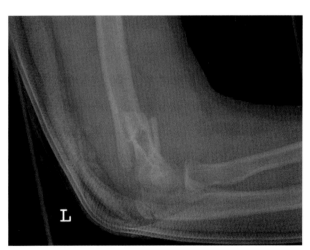

Figure 5.

Radiology findings

There is a distal humerus comminuted fracture, with intra-articular extension. Both columns of the humerus appear to be involved. The radial head appears adequately positioned.

Answers

1. Displaced T-type intra and supracondylar fracture of the distal humerus. In general terms this is an unstable C-type intra-articular fracture.

2. This injury is usually a flexion injury (rare in children, because most elbow injuries in children are extension injuries as the child lands onto an outstretched hand). In this case, the patient lands onto the elbow with the elbow in flexion, most likely landing on the olecranon. The force of the fall is transmitted through the olecranon, up the trochlea and into the distal humerus. The trochlea can get jammed up against the coronoid fossa, which splits the trochlea in half and transmits the force up the distal humerus splitting the medial and lateral condyles, creating the T-type injury as the two columns are separated.

3. This injury should be differentiated from an elbow dislocation or extra-articular supra-condylar humeral fracture. A CT scan will be required to define the injury correctly before surgery.

Management

The gold standard of management is open reduction with internal fixation (ORIF) to restore the articular surface and stabilize the distal humerus. Commonly, an olecranon osteotomy is used for full access to the joint to visualize the reconstruction. Occasionally the fracture can be seen well enough and the olecranon preserved. Today, stabilization is commonly performed with specific plating systems designed for the distal humerus. Stable fixation with an active range of motion can begin immediately and generally a good range of motion can be predicted.

Key points

◆ T-condylar fractures involve both columns of the humerus, always requiring open reduction and internal fixation.

◆ T-condylar fractures are often confused with elbow dislocations or supracondylar humerus fractures.

References

1. Kasser JR, Beaty JH. Supracondylar fractures of the distal humerus. In: *Rockwood and Wilkins' Fractures in Children*, 5th ed. Beaty JH, Kasser JR, Eds. Philadelphia, PA: Lippincott Williams and Wilkins, 2001: 577-624.

2. Otsuka NY, Kasser JR. Supracondylar fractures of the humerus in children. *J Am Acad Orthop Surg* 1997; 5: 19-26.

3. Re PR, Waters PM, Hresko T. T-condylar fractures of the distal humerus in children and adolescents. *J Pediatr Orthop* 1999; 19: 313-8.

4. Papavasilou VA, Beslikas TA. T-condylar fractures of the distal humeral condyles during childhood: an analysis of six cases. *J Pediatr Orthop* 1986; 6: 302-5.

5. Chambers HG, Beaty JH, Kasser JR. Fractures of the proximal radius and ulna. In: *Rockwood and Wilkins' Fractures in Children*, 5th ed. Beaty JH, Kasser JR, Eds. Philadelphia, PA: Lippincott Williams and Wilkins, 2001.

Case 3

Clinical presentation

A three-year-old boy falls off his tricycle onto his left outstretched arm. He presents to the ER the day following the injury, as his mother noted swelling on the outside of his elbow. The patient is also now complaining of elbow pain and not using his arm despite icing and resting it overnight.

Physical examination

There is swelling over the lateral distal humerus, and tenderness over the lateral condyle There is pain and splinting of the elbow with attempted extension. The patient has difficulty with elbow range of motion. Distally, there are no neurovascular deficits.

Review the images below [Figures 6 and 7]. Describe your findings.

Questions

1. What is the diagnosis?

2. What is the mechanism of injury?

3. What is the Jakob classification system?

4. What are the stages of displacement of the injury?

5. What determines the amount of future displacement?

6. What are other associated injuries within the elbow?

7. What is the main problem with assessment of this injury?

8. What are some of the complications of this injury?

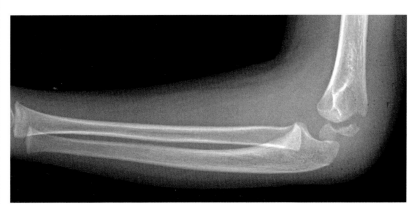

Figure 6.   **Figure 7.**

Radiology findings

There is a fracture of the lateral condyle with dorsal angulation. There is also soft tissue swelling.

Answers

1. Displaced lateral condyle fracture of the elbow.

2. There are two mechanisms described:
    i) push-off theory: the transmission of axial load from the radial head to the lateral condyle that occurs as a child falls onto an outstretched hand, with the hand in its extended valgus position during a fall, allows the radial head to directly impact the lateral condyle and push it off the distal humerus;
    ii) pull-off theory: an avulsion injury that occurs as the lateral condyle is pulled off by the extensor tendons in a varus stress, such as occurs in a fall with the forearm extended and supinated.

3. The Jakob classification system describes the amount of displacement in these fractures, and aids in management:
    i) Stage I: minimally displaced lateral condyle fracture but the joint surface appears intact;
    ii) Stage II: moderately displaced lateral condyle fracture but there may be some lateral translation of the proximal radius and ulna;
    iii) Stage III: completely displaced lateral condyle fragment with elbow instability.

4. In the first stage, the lateral condyle fracture fragment is minimally displaced and the cartilage attaching it to the joint surface is intact, therefore, the joint surface is intact. In the second stage, the fracture goes through the articular surface of the cartilage, which involves the lateral crista of the trochlea. This can create an unstable elbow joint. In the third stage, the lateral condyle is completely displaced, the joint surface is completely disrupted, and since the lateral crista of the trochlea is no longer intact, this allows the proximal radius and ulna to shift posterolaterally and create a valgus deformity.

5. Factors that determine the amount of future displacement of a lateral condyle fracture are the extent of involvement of the trochlear articular cartilage, and the unopposed pull of the extensor muscle mass which is directly attached to the fragment. Although the patient may present to the ER with a large amount of swelling (indicating a greater amount of soft tissue injury), X-rays may show minimal displacement of the fracture. However, the child still has a high risk of having an unstable injury that may be found to be displaced on follow-up radiographs as the swelling decreases.

6. Other associated injuries include fracture of the radial head, elbow dislocation and olecranon fractures.

7. The main problem with assessment of this injury is the difficulty understanding the injury radiographically in the skeletally immature elbow. In the younger child, the only sign may be a change in the shape of the displaced capitellar epiphysis. It is important to be aware of a swollen, painful elbow. If there is any confusion or doubt, an X-ray of the contralateral elbow should be obtained for comparison.

8. Complications include lateral condyle spur deformity, non-union, and cubitus valgus. The latter can classically lead to a tardy ulnar nerve palsy. Late radiographic changes include the fishtail deformity. Two types can present:
    i) angular fishtail deformity, which is thought to result from the gap between the lateral humeral condylar physis and the medial trochlear physis. This deformity usually causes little functional limitation;
    ii) fishtail deformity associated with osteonecrosis of the medial trochlea.

Management

Minimally displaced fractures can be treated non-operatively by placement of the child in a long arm cast. The child should be followed closely to monitor for any radiographic evidence of displacement. Patients are usually kept in a cast for three weeks, followed by a range of motion exercises.

Displaced fractures require anatomic reduction and pinning to avoid displacement caused by the extensor muscle mass. The lateral Kocher approach to the elbow can be used, and pins or screws inserted to hold the reduction. Patients are then casted. If pins are present they are removed at three weeks when the cast is removed. Screws cannot be placed across a growing epiphysis.

Key points

- Lateral condyle fractures are classified according to the Jakob classification system. All fractures with significant displacement should be treated operatively.

- Complications include cubitus valgus deformity, elbow instability, osteonecrosis of the medial trochlea, and late ulnar nerve palsy.

- Displaced fractures are usually treated with anatomic reduction and percutaneous pinning.

References

1. Kasser JR, Beaty JH. Supracondylar fractures of the distal humerus. In: *Rockwood and Wilkins' Fractures in Children*, 5th ed. Beaty JH, Kasser JR, Eds. Philadelphia, PA: Lippincott Williams and Wilkins, 2001: 577-624.

2. Otsuka NY, Kasser JR. Supracondylar fractures of the humerus in children. *J Am Acad Orthop Surg* 1997; 5: 19-26.

3. Skaggs DL. Elbow fractures in children: diagnosis and treatment. *J Am Acad Orthop Surg* 1997; 5: 303-12.

4. Milch H. Fractures and fracture dislocations of humeral condyles. *J Trauma* 1964; 4: 592-607.

5. Badelon O, Bensahel H, Mazda K. Lateral humeral condylar fractures in children: a report of 47 cases. *J Pediatr Orthop* 1988; 8(1): 31-4.

Case 4

Clinical presentation

A 20-month-old girl is brought to the ER by her mother. She reports that her daughter tripped over a rug the day prior to presentation. Immediately after the fall, she was difficult to console and was not using her right hand. The mother iced it, and tried to keep her daughter comfortable. But she reports that today the child is still not using her right hand. Her daughter presents for further evaluation.

Physical examination

The child is sitting comforably in her mother's lap. Her right wrist is in a sling, and she is holding on to her mother with her left hand. The child begins to cry when you take the right arm out of the sling. She cries even more when you push on her distal right forearm and pulls her hand away. The remainder of the exam is difficult because the child is anxious and she will not let you touch her. You manage to palpate good radial and ulnar pulses, you note that the skin over the area of injury is intact, and that there is no gross deformity, swelling or ecchymosis. Her mother reports that she has seen the child move her fingers, but she has not been moving the wrist.

Review the images below [Figures 8 and 9]. Describe your findings.

Questions

1. What is the diagnosis?

2. What is the mechanism of injury?

3. In what age group are these fractures seen?

4. Which bones are commonly involved?

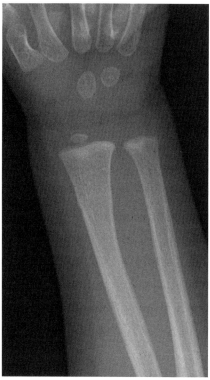

Figure 8.

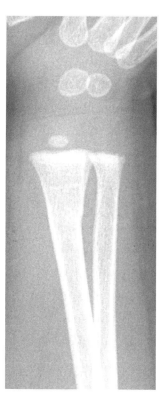

Figure 9.

Radiology findings

Plain films show a cortical irregularity at the distal right radial metaphysis consistent with buckling of the cortex secondary to a compression fracture. A discrete fracture line is not seen. Imaging findings are subtle, showing only a slight irregularity in the cortex.

Answers

1. Torus (buckle) fracture.

2. The most common mechanism of injury is a fall onto an outstretched hand. During bone growth, the area of transition from metaphyseal bone to diaphyseal bone is often the weaker bone, and axial loading during the fall can cause a compression type injury that is a buckle fracture.

3. These fractures are most commonly seen in children between the ages of 5 and 11.

4. The distal metaphysis of the radius and ulna are most frequently affected.

Management

This is a stable fracture with minimal cortical disruption. The child's arm should be immobilized to allow for pain control, promote healing, and prevent futher injury. These injuries can usually be placed in a short arm cast. However, the child is young, and younger children are more apt to wiggle out of their casts. Therefore, this child can be placed in a long arm cast, with the elbow flexed to 90°. The patient can be seen with repeat X-rays in three weeks, the cast invariably removed, and the patient is then allowed to return to normal activities without the need for further immobilization.

Key points

- A torus (buckle) fracture is a compression fracture most commonly involving the distal metaphysis of the radius or ulna.
- Imaging findings are subtle, but reveal cortical irregularity without a discrete fracture line.
- Management includes immobilization for protection only.

References

1. Chambers H, De la Garza JF, O'Brien E, et al. Fractures of the radius and ulna. In: Fractures in Children, Vol. 3. Rockwood CA, Wilkins KE, Beaty JH, Eds. Philadelphia, PA: Lippincott-Raven, 1996: 3: 481-3.

2. Reed MH. Fractures and dislocations of the extremities in children. J Trauma 1977; 17: 351-4.

3. O'Brien ET. Fractures of the hand and wrist region. In: Fractures in Children, 3rd ed. Rockwood CA, Wilkins KE, King RE, Eds. Philadephia, PA: JB Lippincott Company, 1991: 380.

Case 5

Clinical presentation

A four-year-old female is brought to the ER by her father. He reports that she fell off the monkey bars at the playground, landing onto an outstretched hand, and started crying in pain, holding her left wrist.

Physical examination

There is swelling of the left wrist and a mild deformity at the distal forearm. The skin is intact, and there is no ecchymosis. She has palpable radial and ulnar pulses. She can abduct her fingers, retropulse her thumb, and make an OK sign, although she does this with difficulty secondary to pain. She reports normal sensation in her left hand thumb web space, small finger, and over the tips of her fingers.

Review the image below [Figure 10]. Describe your findings.

Questions

1. What is the diagnosis?

2. What is the mechanism of injury?

3. How are these injuries different from a torus (buckle) fracture?

4. What are the acceptable degrees of angulation for this child?

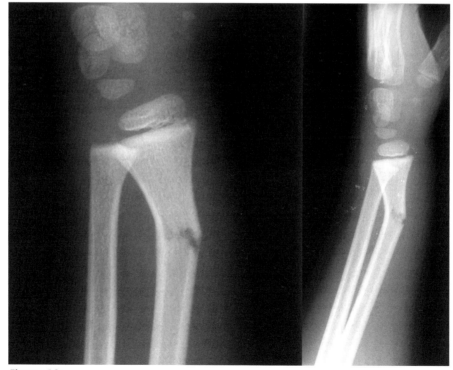

Figure 10.

Radiology findings

There is an incomplete fracture line at the distal radius, with dorsal angulation of the distal fracture fragment. The apex of the fracture points volarly. The cortex and periosteum on the concave side are intact, whereas the cortex and periosteum on the convex side are fractured. There is resultant bowing of the radius. There are no fractures of the ulna.

Answers

1. Greenstick fracture of the distal radius.

2. Greenstick fractures usually occur due to direct trauma, often after a fall onto the outstretched hand. They are a combination of a compressive force, where there is compression of one cortex, and a tension force which causes a fracture through the opposite cortex.

3. A torus (buckle) fracture is a metaphyseal compression fracture without the tension failure on the opposite side. A greenstick fracture

occurs as the next stage of injury, as described above [Figure 11].

4. Young children have a great ability to remodel bone, and for various age groups there are degrees of fracture angulation that are acceptable that will still allow the bone to remodel without residual deformity (Table 2). For patients under five years of age, the acceptable degree of angulation in the sagittal plane is 10-35°. These degrees of angulation also depend on the amount of skeletal maturity. If the patient has a chronologic age of ten years, and/or it appears that the physes on X-ray are close to maturity, then less angulation is acceptable because physiologically there is less potential for remodeling.

Table 2. Degrees of fracture angulation.

Age	Degree of acceptable angulation (sagittal plane)
<5	10-35°
5-10	10-25°
>10	5-20°

Management

The usual indication for manipulation is the presence of a visible deformity. This fracture can be reduced closed. To obtain near anatomic alignment, often the fracture has to be completed to maintain the reduction. In this case, the patient should be consciously sedated. The cortex is intact dorsally, so force should be applied to the wrist in the volar and then again in the dorsal direction to complete the fracture. When using the C-arm, it is important to ensure the bone fragment is aligned in both AP and lateral planes. The patient should be placed in a long arm cast. Bivalving the cast to accomodate for swelling in fractures where a reduction has been performed should always be considered. The patient can be seen in follow-up after a week to confirm maintenance of position. The cast should stay on for 3-4 weeks, at which point if adequate healing is noted on radiographs, the cast can be removed and a range of motion begun.

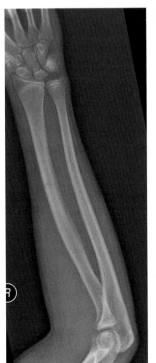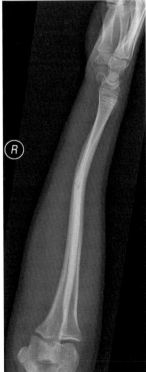

Figure 11. Two views of the right forearm in this 15-year-old patient demonstrate a greenstick injury.

Key points

- Greenstick fractures are seen in children and occur due to direct trauma.
- They are incomplete fractures of a long bone, with disruption of the cortex on one side and deformity on the other side. They are tension-compression injuries.
- Usually to obtain adequate reduction, the fracture needs to be completed.
- For each age group, there are acceptable degrees of angulation that will allow the bone to remodel completely. The older the patient, the less the amount of angulation is acceptable.
- Despite the potential for remodeling, patients with visible deformity are best treated by manipulation.

References

1. Beaty JH, Kasser JR, Eds. *Rockwood and Wilkins' Fractures in Children.* Philadelphia, PA: Lippincott Williams & Wilkins, 2006: 370-2.
2. Koval KJ, Zuckerman JD. *Handbook of Fractures,* 3rd ed. Philadelphia, PA: Lippincott Williams & Wilkins, 2006.

Case 6

Clinical presentation

A 12-year-old girl falls off a trampoline landing on her left hand. She immediately has pain in her left forearm, and notes that instead of being straight, it is now S-shaped. She presents to the ER for further evaluation.

Physical examination

There is gross deformity of the forearm. There is swelling near the distal forearm, but the skin is intact. The patient has palpable radial and ulnar pulses. She can abduct her fingers, retropulse her thumb, and make an OK sign, but she does this with difficulty due to pain. Sensation is intact to light touch in the radial, median, and ulnar nerve distributions. The patient is unwilling to allow you to move her wrist.

Review the images below [Figures 12 and 13]. Describe your findings.

Questions

1. What is the diagnosis?

2. What is the mechanism of injury?

3. What degree of angulation is acceptable?

4. During fixation, what is one of the more critical measures of displacement to be wary of?

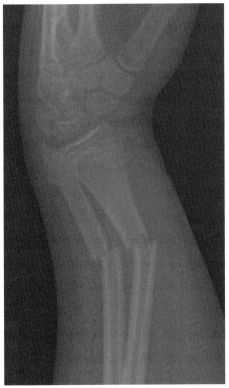

Figure 12.

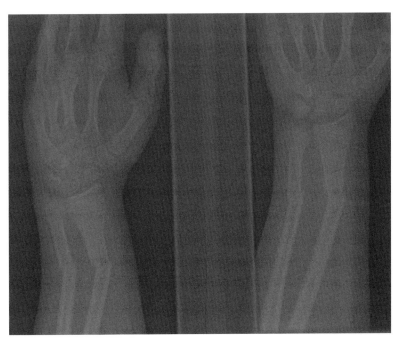

Figure 13.

Radiology findings

There are transverse fractures of the proximal distal third radius and ulna diaphysis, with apex volar angulation. There is minimal translation in the AP plane.

Answers

1. Complete both bone forearm fracture of the distal one third shafts of the radius and ulna in a child.

2. Most of these injuries result from an axial load onto the extremity, combined with a rotational component around the wrist. This causes the break to occur in the forearm, with angulation.

3. The potential for remodeling during the healing process allows a residual angulation to be acceptable as it will grow straight with time. The remodeling capacity depends on the amount of remaining growth the child has and the specific anatomy of the deformity. Degrees of acceptable angulation vary per age group. In addition, many children, who have a physiologic age younger than their chronologic age, can tolerate more angulation. In general, however, the older a child is and the further away the fracture is from the physes, the less remodeling potential is available. In patients younger than eight years old, approximately 20° of angulation and bayonet apposition can be accepted. In those older than eight years old, the limit is much less, with only approximately 10° of angulation, and less than a centimeter of shortening. In practical terms a visible deformity is still rarely acceptable. A good rule is to correct the position by manipulation if the deformity is visible.

4. Aside from translation and angulation in the AP and lateral planes, there is also a rotational deformity in this fracture pattern. Rotational malalignment does not often correct itself fully through remodeling, and for this reason, the older the child, the greater importance it is that rotation be accurately corrected. In general for every degree of malrotation of the fracture fragment, there is approximately a 1-2° loss in forearm pronation and supination. This can cause significant functional limitations.

Management

The fracture should be initially reduced in the ER and a cast applied [Figure 14]. If acceptable alignment is obtained in all planes, then the patient can be followed radiographically (usually at a week) to confirm that the reduction is maintained. If reduction is lost, operative reduction and fixation should be considered.

ER reduction is performed under conscious sedation. To reduce the fracture correctly, rotation, AP translation, and angulation all need to be corrected. A combination of traction, increasing the deformity to disengage fragments followed by correction may be required. In general with apex volar deformities, the forearm should be pronated and with apex dorsal, supinated. After reduction, X-rays are taken to ensure acceptable alignment using the guidelines above. This is a 12-year-old child, so 10° of angulation is the

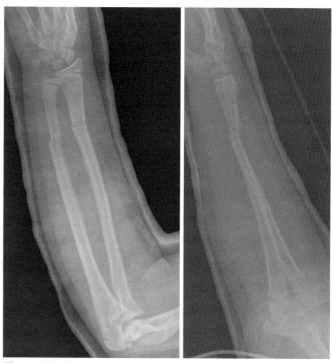

Figure 14. Post-reduction X-rays show minimal translation on the AP plane, and decreased angulation on the lateral X-ray to less than 10°. The lateral X-ray also shows the cortices of the radius and ulna lining up without abnormal rotation of the hand. From this it can be postulated that there is minimal residual rotational deformity of the forearm fracture.

maximum acceptable, with minimal rotational deformity. If an appropriate reduction is obtained, the patient is placed in a long arm cast with the elbow flexed at 90°. This is to prevent additional rotation at the elbow which may displace the reduction. The cast can be bivalved if there is a concern for swelling. The patient is then followed radiographically to ensure the reduction is maintained.

Should the reduction be lost on follow-up, there are several options including remanipulation or operative fixation (both flexible nails or plating techniques are possibilities).

Key points

♦ Both bone forearm fractures have an axial load as well as a rotational component that cause the fracture.

♦ Rotation is the least likely to remodel appropriately in a child, and careful attention should be paid to this component during reduction.

♦ For children less than eight years of age, roughly 20° of angulation and bayonet apposition is acceptable. For over eight years of age, 10° of angulation and less than 1cm of shortening are acceptable.

♦ Manipulation is performed to correct a visible deformity.

♦ If appropriate reduction is obtained, these fractures can be managed non-operatively.

References

1. Birkbeck DP, Failla JM, Hoshaw SJ. The interosseous membrane affects load distribution in the forearm. *J Hand Surg [Am]* 1997; 22(6): 975-80.

2. Hollister AM, Gellman H, Waters RL. The relationship of the interosseous membrane to the axis of rotation of the forearm. *Clin Orthop* 1994; (298): 272-6.

3. Wyrsch B, Mencio GA, Green NE. Open reduction and internal fixation of pediatric forearm fractures. *J Pediatr Orthop* 1996; 16(5): 644-50.

Case 7

Clinical presentation

A 13-year-old gymnast presents to the ER with two days of left groin pain. She noted the onset of pain after her gymnastics practice, thought she had pulled a muscle, and iced the area. She is able to walk. Her pain has not improved, and she is brought in by her coach after her inability to perform at practice.

Physical examination

The patient has no gross deformity of her left hip. She has some tenderness just above her hip joint. Her pain is recreated with hip flexion and knee extension. Distally, she has no neurovascular deficits.

Review the image below [Figure 15]. Describe your findings.

Questions

1. What is the diagnosis?

2. What is the mechanism of injury?

3. In what group of patients are these injuries most commonly seen?

4. What other differential diagnoses should be considered?

5. Where else in the pelvis can this type of injury be seen?

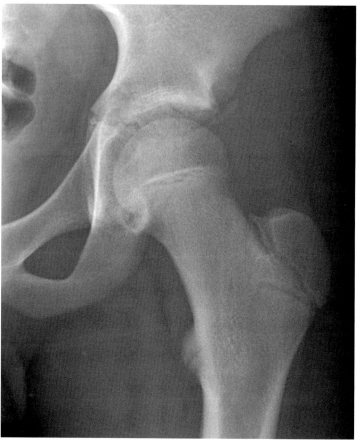

Figure 15.

Radiology findings

There is a minimally displaced bone fragment at the left anterior inferior iliac spine, consistent with an avulsion fracture. There are no other identified fractures or evidence of a left hip dislocation.

Answers

1. Avulsion fracture at the anterior inferior iliac spine (AIIS).

2. An avulsion fracture at the anterior inferior iliac spine results from sudden, forceful traction of the rectus femoris muscle. This can happen during intense physical activity, such as during a gymnastics practice, running or during kicking sports such as soccer and rugby.

3. These injuries almost exclusively occur in young adolescent athletes and usually occur with the hip hyperextended and the knee flexed.

4. This avulsed fragment must be differentiated from an os acetabuli or acetabular epiphysis. This can be done by obtaining comparative X-rays of the contralateral hip to verify that the avulsed fragment is an abnormal finding and not an additional center of ossification.

5. In the pelvis, avulsion fractures are also commonly seen at two other apophyses, the anterior superior iliac spine (ASIS) [Figure 16] and the ischial tuberosity [Figure 17]. The sartorius muscle originates at the anterior superior iliac spine, and the hamstring muscles and hip adductors attach at the ischial tuberosity (see Table 3 for various muscle function). As with avulsion fractures at the AIIS, these are also seen in adolescent athletic patients.

Table 3. Muscle function around the pelvis.

Muscle	Origin	Attachment	Function	Innervation
Sartorius	ASIS	Medial tibia	Flexes the hip, externally rotates knee	Femoral n.
Rectus femoris	AIIS	Tibial tubercle via the patellar tendon	Hip flexion, knee extension	Femoral n.
Adductor magnus	Ischiopubic ramus /ischial tuberosity	Linea aspera and adductor tubercle	Adducts the hip	Posterior division of the obturator n., and sciatic n.
Biceps femoris	Ischial tuberosity (long head), linea aspera (short head)	Head of the fibula	Hip extension, knee flexion	Sciatic n.
Semitendinosus	Ischial tuberosity	Anterior medial tibia	Hip extension, knee flexion	Sciatic n.
Semimembranosus	Ischial tuberosity	Posterior of medial condyle of tibia	Hip extension, knee flexion	Sciatic n.

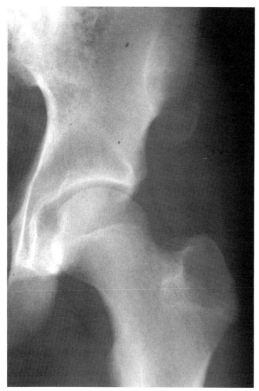

Figure 16. Avulsion fracture at the left anterior superior iliac spine (ASIS).

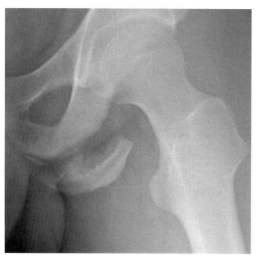

Figure 17. Avulsion fracture at the left ischial tuberosity.

Management

These injuries can be managed non-operatively. The patient should avoid aggravating activity for approximately three weeks and have protected weight bearing on crutches. The patient should be totally asymptomatic with healing on X-rays before return to sport activities is considered. On occasion, large symptomatic bony prominences at the site of the avulsion may cause irritation and may need removal. Significant avulsions of the ischium can cause difficulty sitting and sciatic nerve problems and may be better managed surgically.

Key points

- These injuries most often occur in active adolescents.
- They are often due to a forceful contraction of the hamstrings, hip adductors, or rectus femoris.
- They can be managed non-operatively.
- Images of the contralateral extremity can be taken to rule out a secondary site of ossification versus a true avulsion injury.
- Other pelvic avulsion injuries should be recognized.

References

1. Beaty JH, Kasser JR, Eds. *Rockwood and Wilkins' Fractures in Children*, 6th ed. Philadelphia, PA: Lippincott Williams & Wilkins, 2006: 839-41.

Case 8

Clinical presentation

A 26-month-old female is brought into the ER by her parents after they had noticed her refusing to walk on her right leg. The parents do not recall a definite history of recent trauma.

Physical examination

On exam, when the child is placed on the ground, she refuses to stand. She touches her left foot to the ground, but not her right. She cries with palpation of her tibial shaft, and does not allow any range of motion at the knee or ankle. She has palpable posterior tibial and dorsalis pedis pulses. Further motor exam is difficult because the child is upset, but according to her parents, she will dorsiflex and plantarflex at the ankle.

Review the image below [Figure 18]. Describe your findings.

Questions

1. What is the diagnosis?

2. What is the mechanism of injury?

3. If the initial radiographs had been negative, what other imaging modality would you consider in cases of high suspicion for this injury?

4. If you are the physician caring for this patient, what important information should you delineate from the history given by the parents?

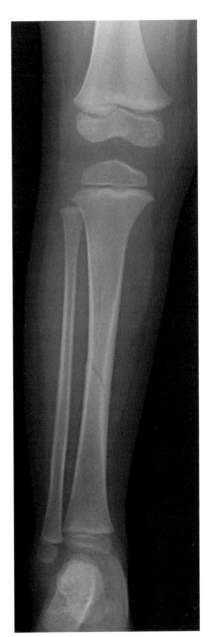

Figure 18.

Radiology findings

On a frontal view of the right tibia and fibula, there is a subtle, non-displaced, oblique fracture of the midshaft of the tibia. It is visualized as a thin lucency. Although difficult to appreciate on the given image, there is mild periosteal reaction adjacent to this lucency on a magnified view.

Answers

1. Toddler's fracture.

2. The cause of the majority of Toddler's fractures is not always a witnessed event. The child usually has had a fall in which there is a sudden twisting or rotational motion of the foot or lower extremity (for example, quickly running on the playground, getting the foot stuck and then falling).

3. In many cases, initial radiographs may be negative for a Toddler's fracture. A follow-up study usually demonstrates a periosteal reaction, or sclerosis at the fracture site, indicating healing. A nuclear bone scintigraphy study can be obtained to further evaluate the presence of a fracture in the situation where radiographs are negative. This will demonstrate increased focal uptake at the fracture site.

4. Spiral or oblique fractures of the midshaft of the tibia may indicate child abuse which should always be suspected. Hence, it is important to carefully obtain a good history from the parents. Toddler's fractures usually occur secondary to falls that are unwitnessed, making it difficult to determine whether non-accidental injury plays a role. In child abuse, there are often injuries outside of the musculoskeletal system, the child may have other multiple skeletal injuries on presentation, or may have a history of treatment for multiple skeletal injuries within a relatively short period of time.

Management

A 26-month-old child has bones with a great potential for remodeling. Therefore, most tibial shaft fractures, both displaced and minimally displaced (as above), can be treated in a long leg cast with the knee bent at 70-90°. Children heal rapidly, and the cast can likely be removed four weeks after injury, at which point the child will be allowed to resume her regular activities. The knee is flexed to 70-90° to prevent weight bearing on the affected limb. Since this is a minimally displaced fracture, there is no need to control rotation of the tibia by casting above the knee. However, an above knee cast is always used in very small children as short leg casts come off too easily.

Key points

◆ Toddler's fractures are common in toddlers and preschoolers and occur due to a sudden twisting/rotational motion of the tibia.

◆ Non-accidental injury must be considered.

◆ Initial films may be negative, or may demonstrate a spiral, non-displaced lucency.

◆ The patients are usually placed in a long leg cast with the knee flexed to 70-90°.

References

1. Dunbar JS, Owen HF, Nogrady MB, et al. Obscure tibial fracture of infants: the toddler's fracture. J Can Assoc Radiol 1964; 15: 136-44.

2. Blumber K, Patterson RJ. The toddler's cuboid fracture. Radiology 1991; 179: 93-4.

Case 9

Clinical presentation

A two-year-old child is brought to the ER by his parents. They report that the child fell down the stairs earlier in the day, and has since been inconsolable and not moving his right leg. They bring their child in for further evaluation.

Physical examination

On exam, there is swelling over the right thigh. The child cries with any attempted hip or knee range of motion. He is most comfortable with his leg resting on a pillow with minimal movement. He refuses to bear weight. Distally, he has palpable pulses, and when the soles of his feet are tickled, he dorsiflexes and plantarflexes his right foot.

Review the images below [Figures 19 and 20]. Describe your findings.

Questions

1. What is the diagnosis?

2. What is the mechanism of injury?

3. What should the physician be wary of in a child that presents with this fracture pattern?

4. Describe the changes in the femur as a child ages.

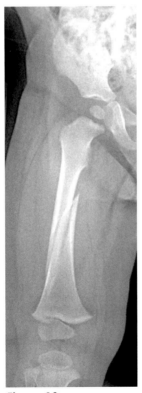

Figure 19.

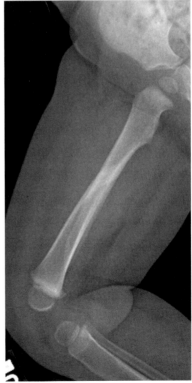

Figure 20.

Radiology findings

There is an oblique/spiral fracture of the femoral shaft in a young child. There is minimum displacement and no shortening.

Answers

1. Oblique/spiral femur fracture.

2. Femur fractures in young children, with the fracture pattern above, are usually due to a twisting/rotational force around the shaft of the femur.

3. With such a fracture pattern, the physician should be wary of child abuse. The clinical history should be carefully recorded and confirmed to be compatible with the observed injury. The child should be fully assessed (often radiographically) for additional injuries. Unexplained or multiple fractures in various stages of healing are signs of abuse, even repeated abuse.

4. As the child grows, there is an increase in femoral shaft diameter and thickness of the cortex. This continues into late adolescence. As a result, younger patients require little force to fracture their femurs due to small shaft diameter and a thin cortex, whereas in adolescents a higher force is required to break the femur. This explains why many young children present with femur fractures after a fall during play or with minor trauma, whereas adolescents present with femur fractures after major trauma, such as in a motor vehicle accident.

Management

Management of femur fractures depends on the child's age and size. The following recommendations need to be considered taking the child's clinical and social situation into account. For very small children less than six months of age, the fracture can be treated in either a Pavlik harness, or a posterior splint if the child will tolerate it. For six months to six years of age, femur fractures can be treated in a spica cast.

For 6-12 years, flexible intramedullary nails or sub-muscular plates can be used. The surgeon will advise the family often based on their own experience and the specific situation of the child and family. Adolescents with femoral fractures are usually treated with sub-muscular plating as they are getting too heavy for flexible nails. Adult treatment with an antegrade intramedullary nail cannot be used until the femoral capital epiphysis has closed because of the rare but devastating potential complication of avascular necrosis of the femoral head. This results from the nail entry site damaging the essential feeder vessels to the femoral head.

In this case, the child is two years old with a minimally displaced fracture, and no associated shortening. The child can be placed in a spica cast and monitored closely. The child is kept in the cast for roughly 6-12 weeks until healing is noted. Afterwards, they are allowed to resume activity as tolerated. Subsequent growth of the femur will almost certainly correct any residual deformity at this age.

Key points

- ◆ The femur changes from a narrow, thin bone in young children, to a wider, thicker bone in adolescents.

- ◆ Higher-energy trauma is required to break a femur in an adolescent.

- ◆ A spiral femur fracture should alert the examiner to the possibility of abuse.

- ◆ Femur fractures are treated according to the age and size of the child. Younger children receive conservative management with casting and harnesses, and older children more invasive methods such as flexible nails and sub-muscular plates.

- ◆ Adult intramedullary nails cannot be used until closure of the capital epiphysis because of increased risk for development of avascular necrosis of the femoral head.

- ◆ Beware missing child abuse in infants presenting with fractures.

References

1. Leventhal JM, Thomas SA, Rosenfield NS, Markowitz RI. Fractures in young children. Distinguishing child abuse from unintentional injuries. *Am J Dis Child* 1993; 147(1): 87-92.

2. Sponseller PD, Beaty JH. Fractures and dislocations about the knee. In: *Fractures in Children*, 4th ed. Philadelphia, PA: Lippincott-Raven, 1996: 1231-329.

3. Beaty JH. Pediatric femur fractures. Presented at the 28th Annual Orthopaedic Fall Seminar, Alfred I duPont Hospital for Children, Wilmington, Delaware, October 3, 1998.

4. Blasier RD, Aronson J, Tursky EA. External fixation of pediatric femur fractures. *J Pediatr Orthop* 1997; 17(3): 342-6.

Appendix

Normal X-rays

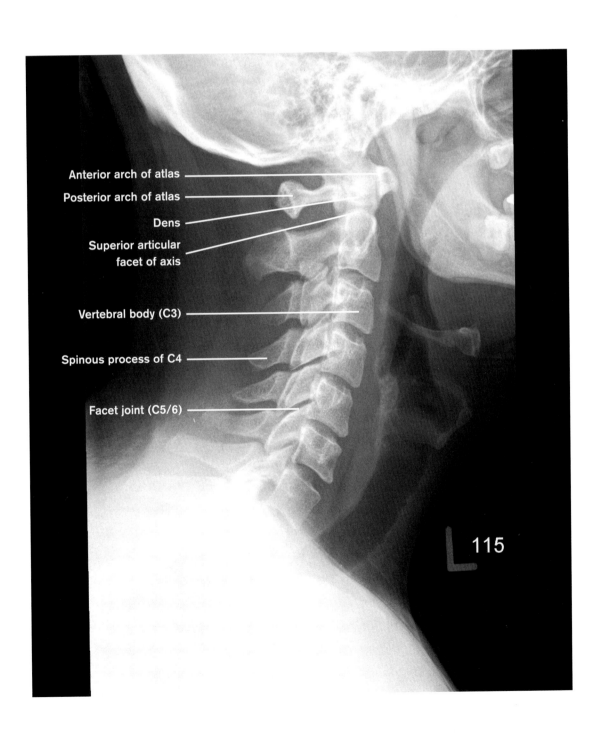

Anterior arch of atlas

Posterior arch of atlas

Dens

Superior articular facet of axis

Vertebral body (C3)

Spinous process of C4

Facet joint (C5/6)

115

Dens

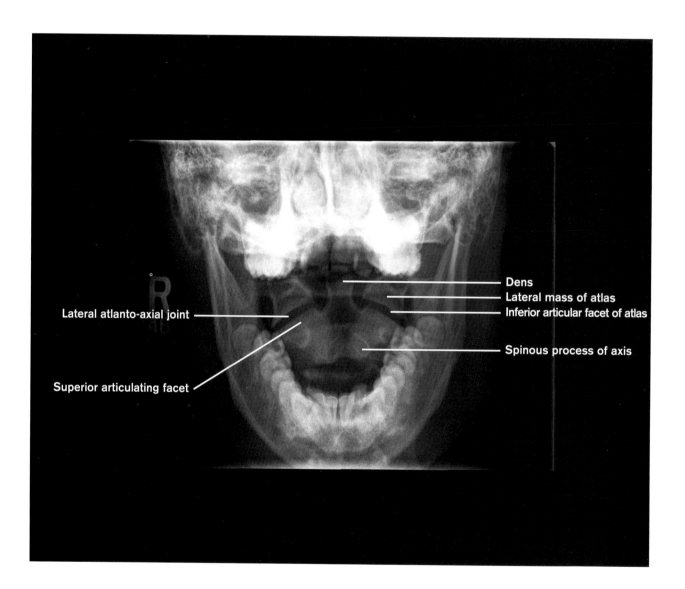

Lateral atlanto-axial joint

Superior articulating facet

Dens

Lateral mass of atlas

Inferior articular facet of atlas

Spinous process of axis

Shoulder

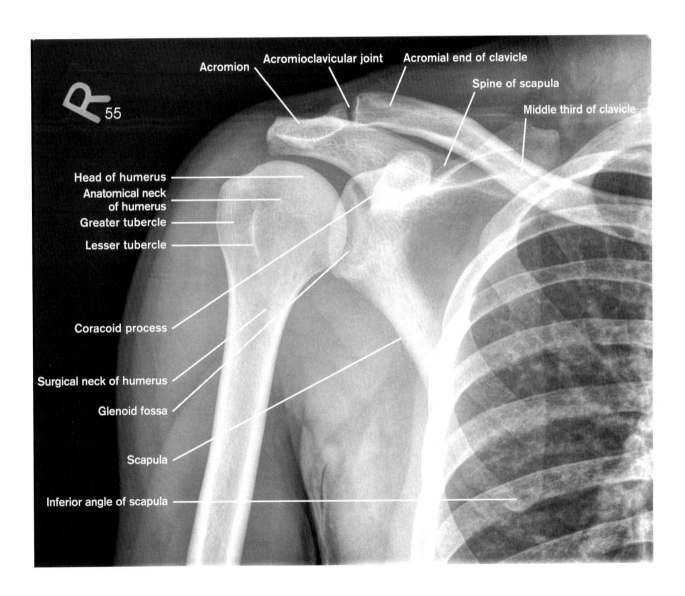

Humerus

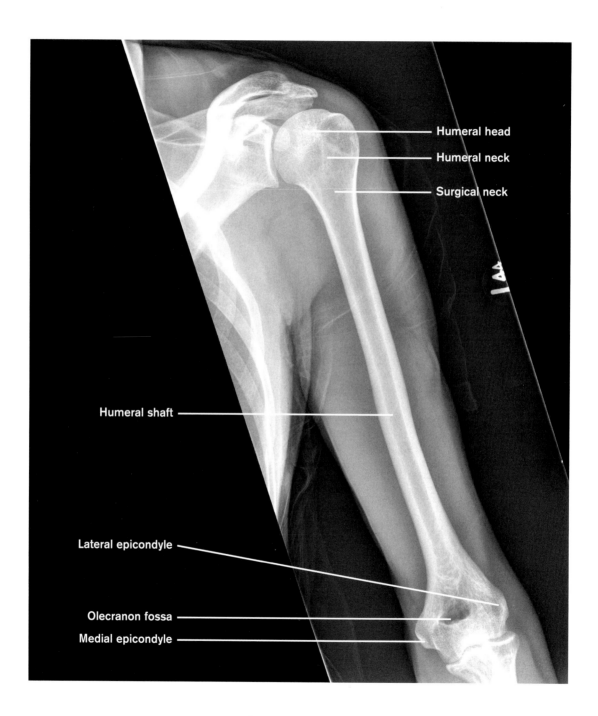

Humeral head

Humeral neck

Surgical neck

Humeral shaft

Lateral epicondyle

Olecranon fossa

Medial epicondyle

Elbow

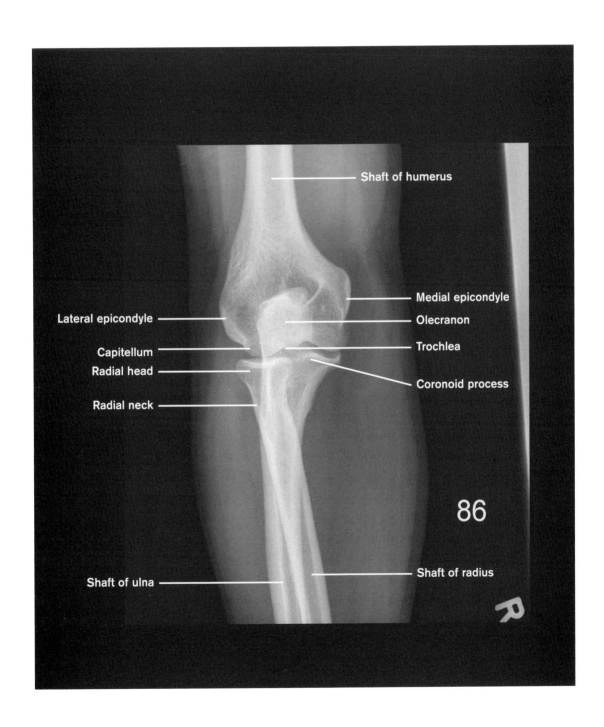

Shaft of humerus

Medial epicondyle

Lateral epicondyle

Olecranon

Capitellum

Trochlea

Radial head

Coronoid process

Radial neck

86

Shaft of radius

Shaft of ulna

Elbow lateral

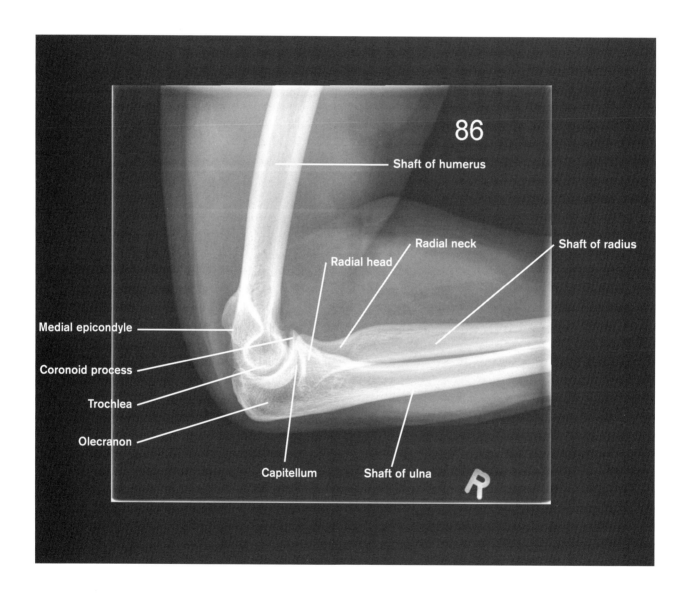

86

Shaft of humerus

Radial neck

Shaft of radius

Radial head

Medial epicondyle

Coronoid process

Trochlea

Olecranon

Capitellum

Shaft of ulna

R

Forearm

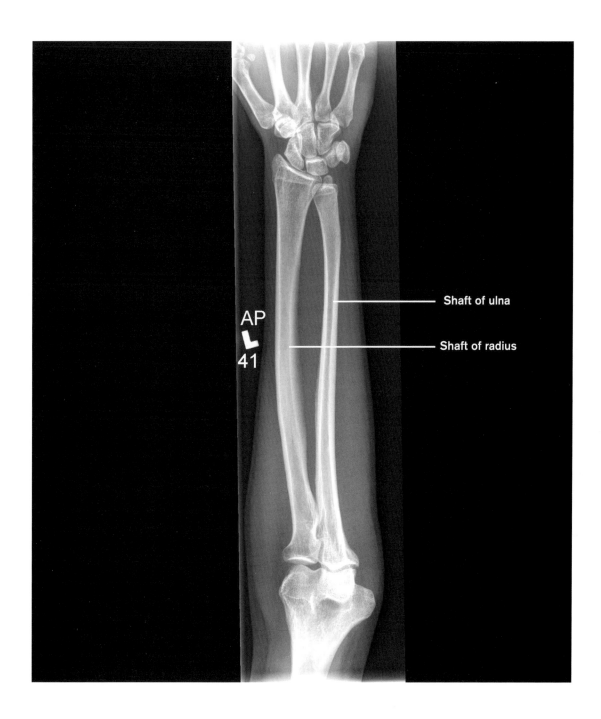

AP
L
41

Shaft of ulna

Shaft of radius

Wrist

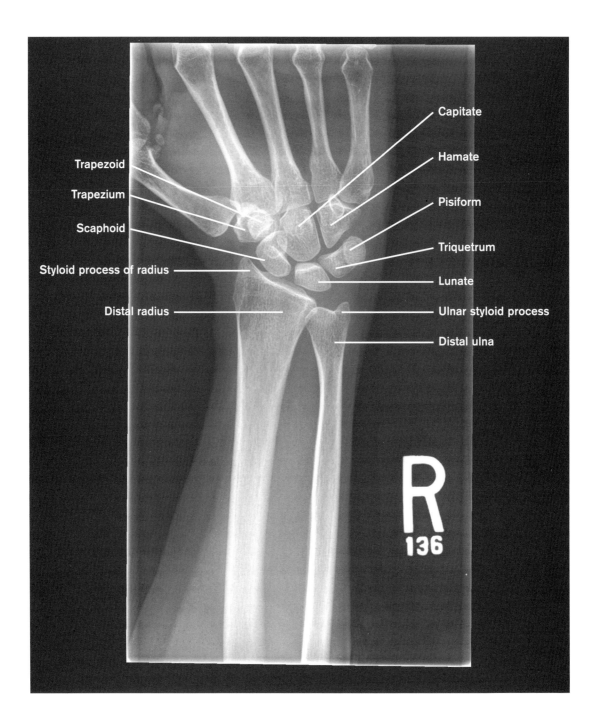

Wrist

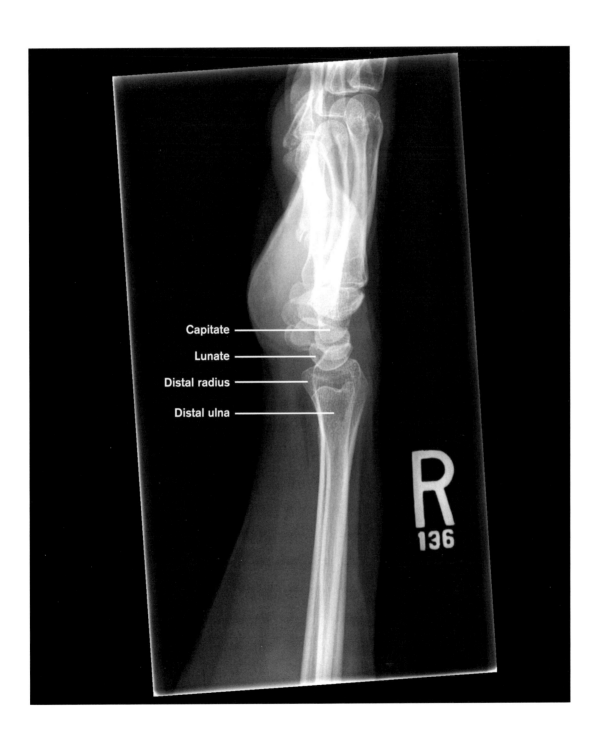

Capitate

Lunate

Distal radius

Distal ulna

Hand

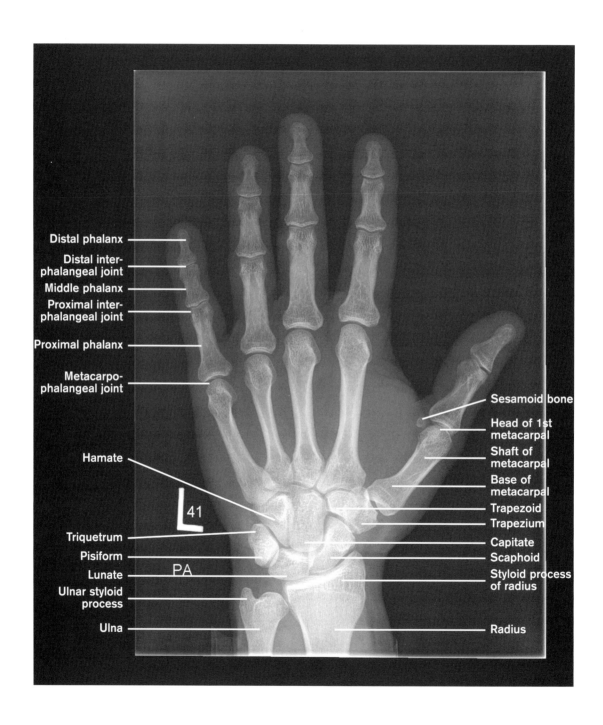

Distal phalanx

Distal inter-phalangeal joint

Middle phalanx

Proximal inter-phalangeal joint

Proximal phalanx

Metacarpo-phalangeal joint

Hamate

Triquetrum

Pisiform

Lunate

Ulnar styloid process

Ulna

Sesamoid bone

Head of 1st metacarpal

Shaft of metacarpal

Base of metacarpal

Trapezoid

Trapezium

Capitate

Scaphoid

Styloid process of radius

Radius

Thoracic spine

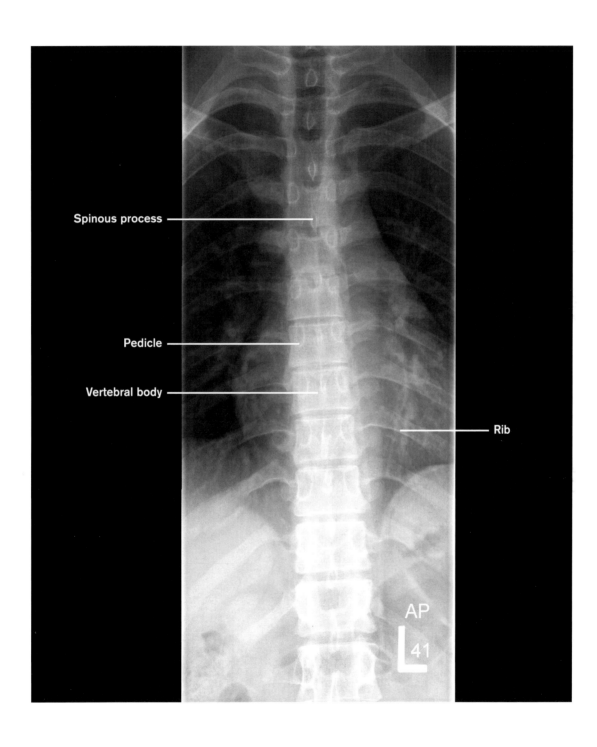

Spinous process

Pedicle

Vertebral body

Rib

AP

Thoracic spine

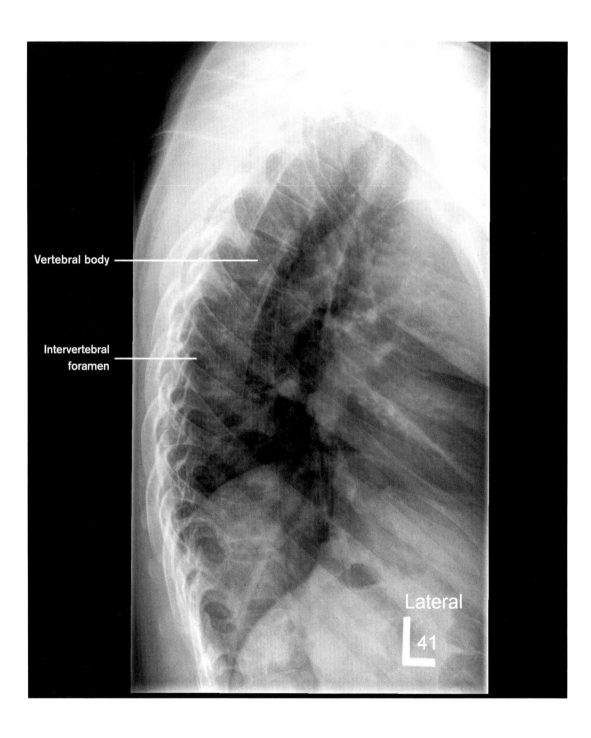

Lumbar spine

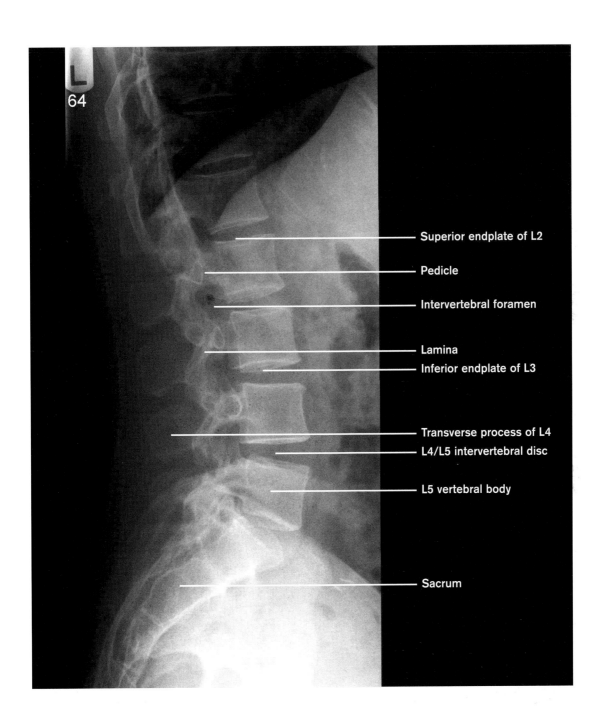

- Superior endplate of L2
- Pedicle
- Intervertebral foramen
- Lamina
- Inferior endplate of L3
- Transverse process of L4
- L4/L5 intervertebral disc
- L5 vertebral body
- Sacrum

Lumbar spine

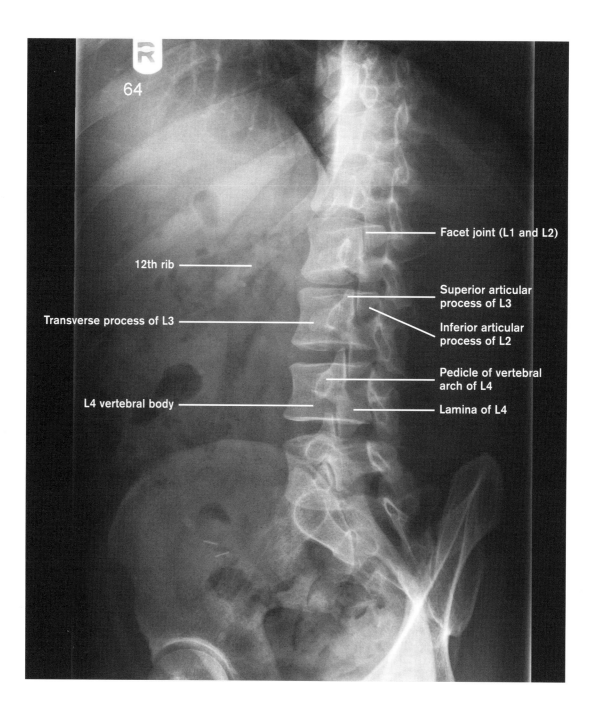

Sacrum

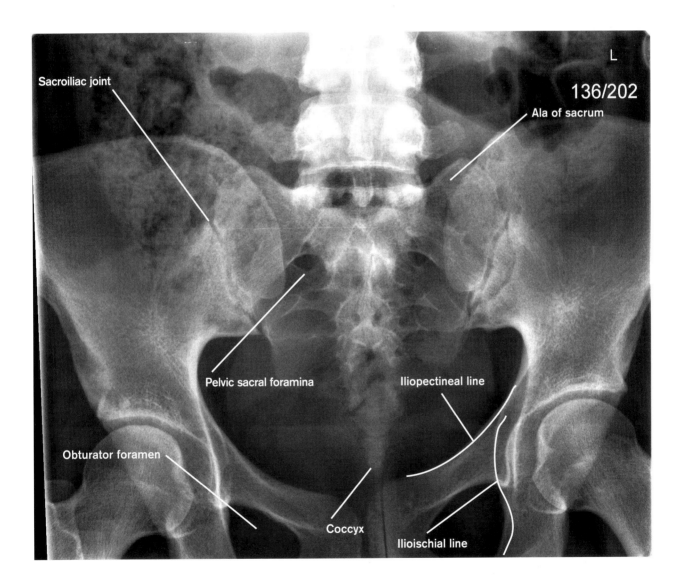

L

136/202

Sacroiliac joint

Ala of sacrum

Pelvic sacral foramina

Iliopectineal line

Obturator foramen

Coccyx

Ilioischial line

Pelvis

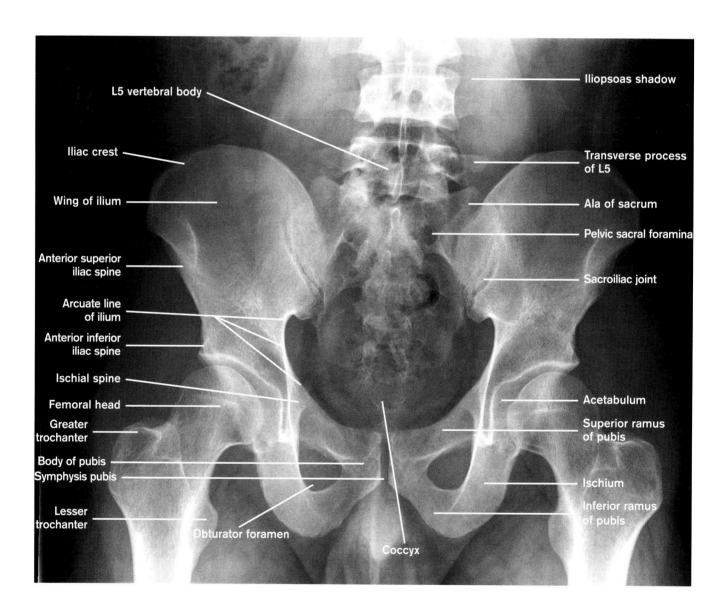

L5 vertebral body

Iliac crest

Wing of ilium

Anterior superior
iliac spine

Arcuate line
of ilium

Anterior inferior
iliac spine

Ischial spine

Femoral head

Greater
trochanter

Body of pubis

Symphysis pubis

Lesser
trochanter

Obturator foramen

Coccyx

Iliopsoas shadow

Transverse process
of L5

Ala of sacrum

Pelvic sacral foramina

Sacroiliac joint

Acetabulum

Superior ramus
of pubis

Ischium

Inferior ramus
of pubis

Hip

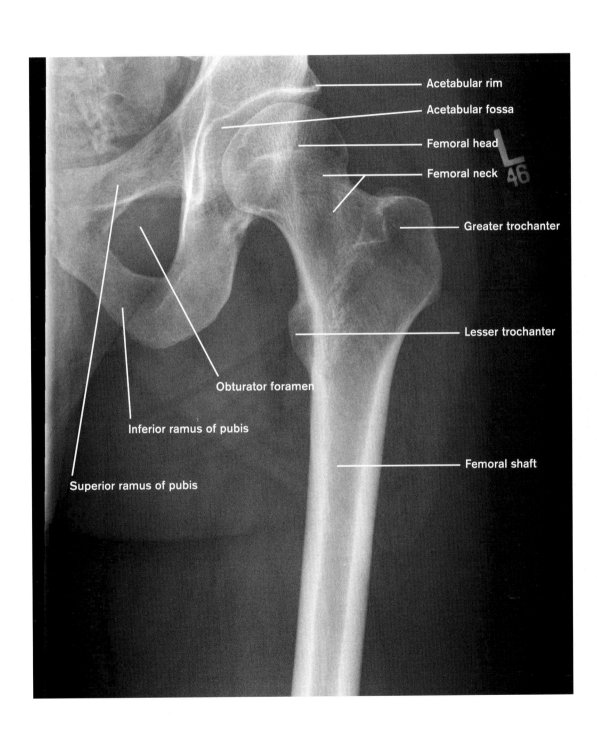

Acetabular rim

Acetabular fossa

Femoral head

Femoral neck

Greater trochanter

Lesser trochanter

Obturator foramen

Inferior ramus of pubis

Femoral shaft

Superior ramus of pubis

Knee

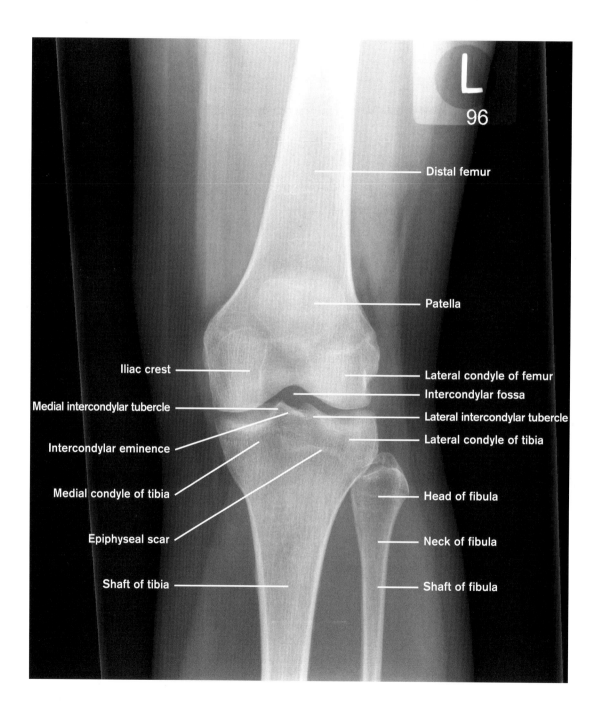

L
96

Distal femur

Patella

Iliac crest

Medial intercondylar tubercle

Intercondylar eminence

Medial condyle of tibia

Epiphyseal scar

Shaft of tibia

Lateral condyle of femur

Intercondylar fossa

Lateral intercondylar tubercle

Lateral condyle of tibia

Head of fibula

Neck of fibula

Shaft of fibula

Lower limb

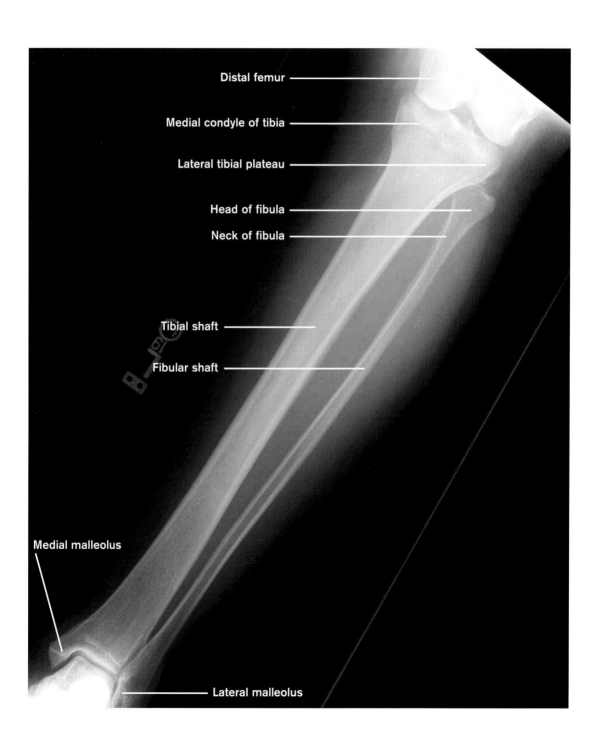

Distal femur

Medial condyle of tibia

Lateral tibial plateau

Head of fibula

Neck of fibula

Tibial shaft

Fibular shaft

Medial malleolus

Lateral malleolus

Ankle

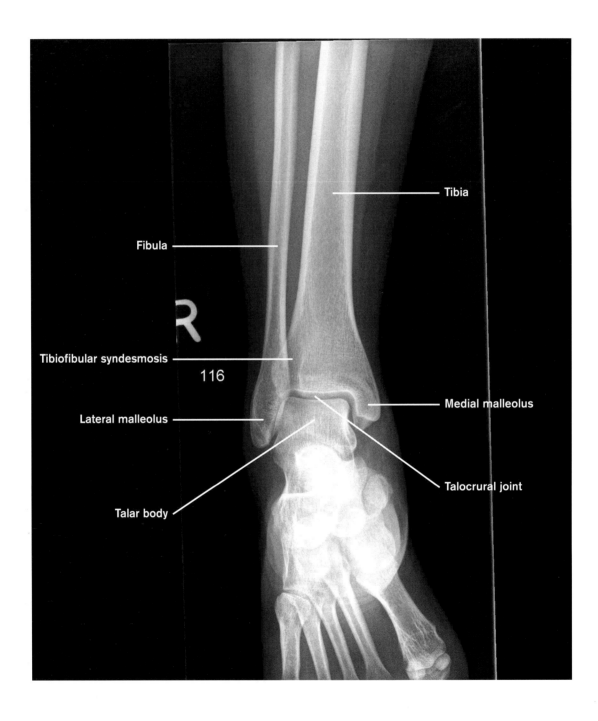

Ankle lateral

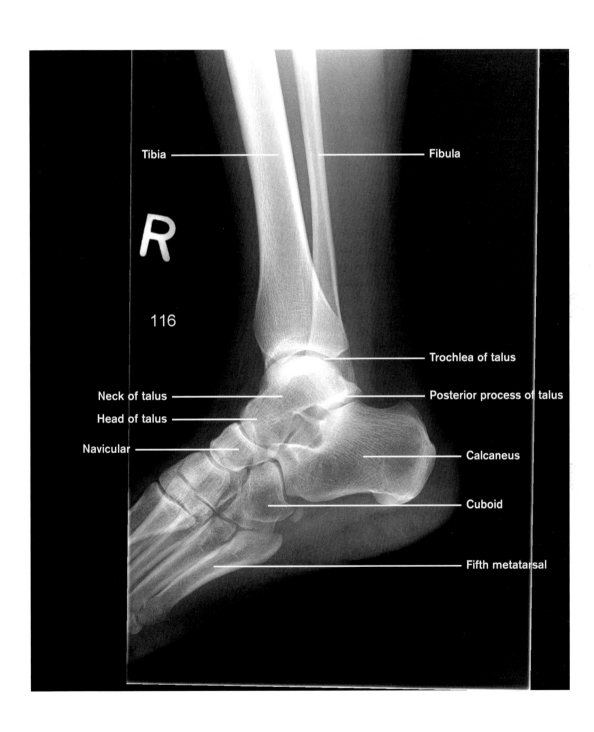

Tibia

Fibula

R

116

Trochlea of talus

Neck of talus

Posterior process of talus

Head of talus

Navicular

Calcaneus

Cuboid

Fifth metatarsal

Foot

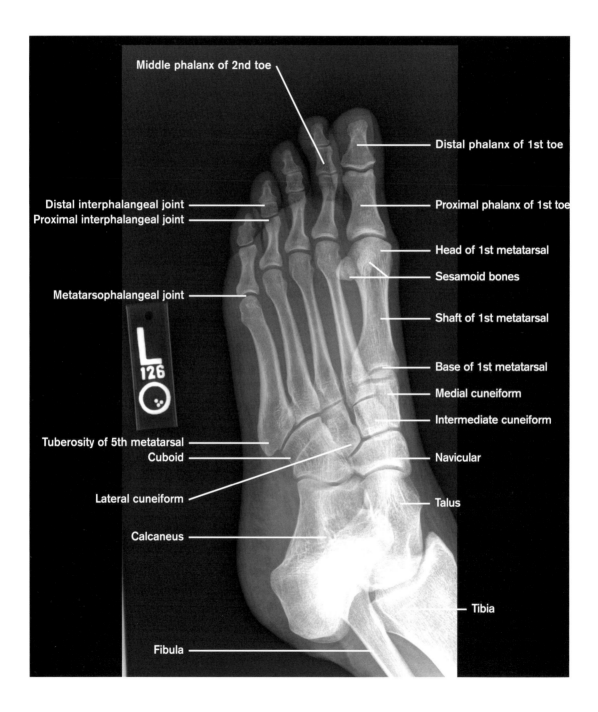

Fracture and injury index

Pages